OPERATION FLIGHT NURSE

Real-Life Medical Emergencies

David M Kaniecki MSN ACNP-C CCRN

Flight Nurse Practitioner

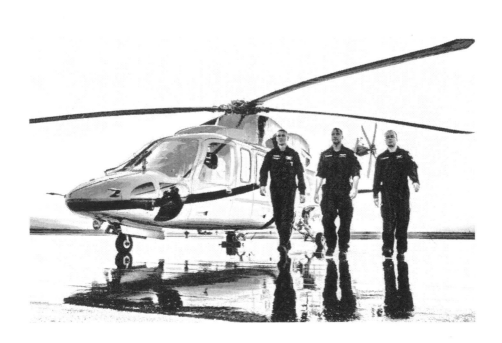

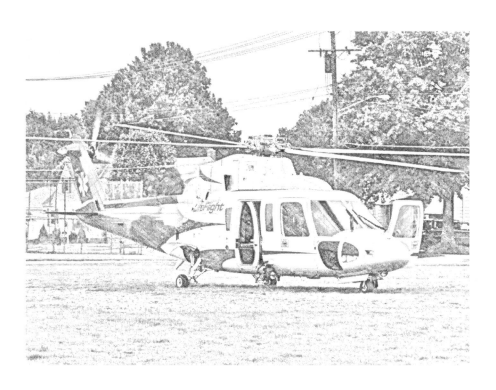

ABOUT THIS BOOK

Life-Flight-Teams are called to transport those in need of critical medical care to an institution capable of managing their condition. On occasion, life-altering events can be prevented from ever occurring, or measures may be taken by both patients and medical providers to reduce the impact these events have. I wrote this book for two reasons, to enlighten those curious about the flight-nurse profession and to share with the public and those new to critical care some take home points from these medical emergencies.

I am asked daily by both the public and those in the healthcare industry about my career as a life-flight nurse. My goal is to answer this question, at least in part, by sharing my more memorable experiences as a life-flight nurse, linking each story to a teachable event. I have tried to explain each medical term initially for the reader but please refer to the *Glossary of Terms* if you do not understand a particular word. Each story, except for the last, follows a basic format.

Format

Setting - the events or patient symptoms leading to the need for emergency transport.

Everyday Language Of What Might Be Going On – an easy to understand, plain language explanation of what is going on medically with the patient.

The Flight Out and Game Plan - my thoughts and plans for the transport and/or events while en route to pick up our patient. Most of the stories are helicopter transports, but a few are by ambulance or fixed wing (i.e. plane).

The Transport - details of the transport with the patient in our care.

The Outcome - when known, patient outcomes during and after the hospital stay.

Take Home Points: - I believe the greatest teaching methods are through real life experiences. I have tried to relate each story to lessons that can be learned from the events. After each story, there is a section designated for *nurses or emergency service (EMS) providers* and one for the *public*. I have learned a great deal throughout my career and hope to share several key lessons with you in easy to understand words.

IMPROVE THIS BOOK

If you are a flight nurse, medic, or M.D. and would like to submit a story for follow-up editions to this book, please email operationflightnurse@gmail.com. I realize treatment recommendations change over time and may vary among providers. If you do not agree with any statements made in this book, please email the discrepancy along with an explanation and current reference.

DISCLAIMER

This book is not intended as a substitute for the medical advice of physicians. The reader should regularly consult a physician in matters relating to his/her health with respect to any symptoms that may require diagnosis or medical attention. Some names and identifying transport details may have been changed to protect the privacy of individuals. I have tried to recreate events, settings and conversations from my memories of them. In order to maintain patient anonymity, I have changed or omitted identifying characteristics and details such as physical properties, age, gender, occupations and hospital locations. Although the author has made every effort to ensure that the information in this book was correct at press time, the author does not assume and hereby disclaims any liability to any party for any loss, damage, or disruption caused by errors or omissions, whether such errors or omissions result from negligence, accident, or any other cause.

CONTENTS

SHOULD WE HAVE DONE CPR?

Setting:

An 85 year old woman with a medical history of diabetes, hypertension, and breast cancer had been ill at home for a week. She felt tired and nauseated, and quit eating because she would vomit after each meal. At first this looked like the flu, but her symptoms persisted and, after a couple days, became worse. Her children persuaded her to see her doctor, but he was on vacation, so they convinced her to go to the emergency department (ED) at a small community hospital.

Once at the hospital, tests showed she had a urinary tract infection. Because of her age and other medical problems, the emergency room physician admitted her for closer monitoring and treatment. She began to feel better after several days of intravenous (IV) antibiotics and her physician decided to finally let her go home. But, only two hours before her scheduled discharge, she unexpectedly became confused.

Words she spoke did not make sense half the time. One minute she knew her name, and the next she would either not speak, or her words were random and disorganized.

Concerned the symptoms might be caused by an ongoing stroke, her physician ordered immediate brain imaging. A computerized tomography (CT) scan showed multiple small strokes in her brain, one of which was actively bleeding.

The radiologist who interpreted the scan notified the physician of the results at once. This hospital could not manage her condition or intervene should the bleeding increase, so he initiated transfer to the closest stroke center and requested a helicopter for rapid transport. The nurse prepared the paperwork needed for transfer, but noticed something very important was missing in the medical record.

There were no advanced directives or documentation of the patient's wishes about advanced life support. During the hospital stay, her family had realized this and recalled several conversations in which their mother stated she did not want to "live like a vegetable". Since everyone expected her to recover, they planned to complete this paperwork once she was better and discharged home.

Everyday Language Of What Might Be Going On:

There are multiple reasons why a person may suddenly become confused. One third of hospitalized elderly patients experience confusion. Medications, electrolyte imbalances, withdrawal from drugs or alcohol, infection, and poor vision or hearing are just a few examples of potential causes. Conditions which alter oxygen to the brain, such as a heart attack or pneumonia, can also alter one's mental status. When a patient becomes confused in the hospital, the most life-threatening conditions must be ruled out promptly. In this case, any number of issues may have caused her symptoms, but a head CT was performed right away to look for a stroke.

Not identifying this promptly can cause serious long term complications.

The chapter in this book on intracranial hemorrhage and subarachnoid hemorrhage further explain this disease. The purpose of this story is to emphasize the importance of having advance health care directives and a power of attorney documented. Health care directives are documents containing a specific set of actions specifying what can, or cannot, be done if one is not competent to make their own medical decisions. These documents inform health care professionals as to what extent life-saving-measures should be provided. A power of attorney is a designated person to make health care decisions should a person be incompetent. The power of attorney is used when medical decisions are not clearly stated in the advanced directive. Advanced directives take precedence over the power of attorney.

Many patients think only a power of attorney is needed, but it's important to have both. A power of attorney may not fully understand someone's wishes, or may allow emotions to influence their decisions. An advanced directive may relieve the stress and anxiety imposed on the power of attorney when end-of-life decisions are needed. By declaring one's own wishes with advance directives, the power of attorney is not forced to make difficult decisions on their behalf. The benefit of having a power of attorney, in addition to advanced directives, is to address topics that might not have been considered when drafting the health care directive.

The Flight Out and Game Plan:

With 2 hours to go before the end of shift, my pager vibrated and we were dispatched to a small community hospital 25 miles from our base. The information relayed to us was that our patient had a small hemorrhagic stroke and was to go to the closest stroke center. The patient reportedly was slightly confused, vital signs normal, and she was on a regular nursing floor.

We transport the majority of our patients from an emergency department (ED) or intensive care unit (ICU) because of their high level of acuity. On the rare occasion we go to the regular nursing floor, the transport is often one of two extremes. It is either very simple because the patient is stable, or incredibly chaotic because the patient just crashed and there was no time for transfer to an ICU. Floor rooms typically have two beds per room, are crowded, and the staff are not accustomed to critical emergencies. This combination increases the chaos when it occurs. Based on the information we received, we anticipated an un-complicated transport. This transport started out that way, but turned chaotic very fast.

The Transport:

We landed, the pilots powered down the aircraft, and I did something I seldom do. I told the pilots they didn't need to accompany us, and we would be right back. Little did I know at the time that I would not be back for a few hours. Pilots often go with the medical crew into the hospital to help carry equipment and lift the patient. Since we had a three-person medical crew and the patient was stable on a regular nursing floor, we did not expect to need help. We unloaded our cot and equipment from the aircraft and security escorted us to the nursing floor.

Once at our patient's room, I peeked in and noticed an elderly woman, quietly sleeping in the bed. Two beds were in this room, but she was the only patient and her bed was furthest from the door. Since her vital signs were normal and it looked as if the transport would be straightforward, my partners and I went to talk with the nurse. The patient's nurse gave us a quick update and said the patient was normal earlier, but when the nurse went to check on her again the patient seemed confused. I asked the nurse about our patient's drug allergies and code status, as I do with every patient, and her response proved important to the rest of the transport.

"Well," the nurse said with a short pause, "that's confusing." She went on to explain that the family thought their mother did not want extreme measures to prolong her life, but were going to fill out the paperwork later. "Well, what does that mean...What does she consider extreme?" I asked. "Would she want CPR...Would she want a breathing tube?" The nurse said she didn't know but was trying to contact the patient's daughter, who was the power of attorney.

Not having an official code status put us in an awkward position. While wanting to respect our patient's wishes, nobody truly understood them, and nothing had been documented. If something went wrong during the transport, we had to assume she wanted everything done. Not acting could lead to serious health consequences for our patient, and failing to offer potentially lifesaving measures might be a liability issue for us. Not expecting our patient would need these measures in flight, we proceeded with the transport, hoping someone might get in contact with the daughter before we left.

After speaking with the nurse for several minutes, we went back to talk with and assess our patient. I walked in the room and whispered her name, and she awoke from her sleep.

Although confused, she was alert enough to say her name and showed no signs of being unstable. When I asked what she thought about flying, and to what extent she might want lifesaving measures, she refused to answer. I tried several times to inquire about her code status, but got nowhere: she said to 'ask her daughter those questions.' Not wanting to delay transfer and not expecting any problems, I finished my assessment and proceeded with the transport while my partner placed her on the transport monitor.

We lifted and secured her to the transport cot and that's when everything started to become chaotic. All of a sudden, our patient had a blank facial stare and appeared to not be breathing. I reached to feel for a pulse, which was thankfully there. Next, I searched for any indication of breathing again, thinking perhaps it was my imagination, but she was not breathing. As my heart began to beat a little faster, I shouted her name and shook her several times, but nothing happened. I thought to myself, *this cannot be happening*. Still not convinced, I double checked again, putting my ear next to her mouth and one hand on her chest to feel for movement, but she absolutely was not breathing. Not having any official documentation, or even verbal confirmation of her code status, we had to place a breathing tube. My partner got everything ready and I positioned to place the tube, but about 30 seconds after the episode began she started breathing again.

Although breathing at this point, she no longer responded to any stimulation and just lay on our cot with a blank stare. I asked the nurse if she had noticed anything like that before our arrival and she responded no. Now we really wanted clarification on which measures to offer if this happened again. I asked the nurse if our patient's physician was in the hospital, and to have him come quickly if available.

The nurse left to call the doc while we re-secured the patient to our cot and began to put away the equipment to place the breathing tube. We were almost ready to leave when the nurse came back in the room and said she updated the doctor, who would be there soon.

The physician walked in 2 or 3 minutes later. He had telephoned the daughter, and said that she and other family members would be at the hospital in 20 minutes. While on the phone, our patient's daughter had conveyed to not transport her mother from that hospital but did not want to make any code decisions until family arrived. The doc asked if we could wait and monitor the patient until the family came and we agreed. Seconds after speaking with the doc, with the patient still on our cot, her symptoms came back.

She stopped breathing again. I yelled her name and shook her body but nothing happened. Five seconds went by...10 seconds...still nothing. She was not breathing but had a pulse. However, if she continued to not breathe this pulse would soon go away. I said to the doc, "We need to do something." We rushed to get the intubation equipment back out and positioned her to place a breathing tube. I placed a mask over her nose and mouth and began to breathe for her with an ambu bag.

"Doc, we can't do this for 20 minutes", I said with the mask over her nose and mouth as I squeezed a breath of air into her lungs. "We need to place a breathing tube. We can always pull it out later." He agreed and I began to place the tube. I opened her mouth, inserted a laryngoscope, and manipulated it to visualize her vocal cords. Her cords came into clear view and I placed the breathing tube into her trachea (windpipe).

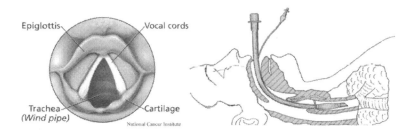

Epiglottis   Vocal cords

Trachea   Cartilage
(Wind pipe)
National Cancer Institute

We verified the tube was in the trachea, and manually ventilated our patient. The family was on their way and we knew we would no longer be transporting the patient, but with a breathing tube in, she could not stay on the regular nursing floor. Only intensive care units or emergency departments are capable of monitoring patients on a mechanical ventilator. A "code blue" had been called during the intubation and there were about 10 people crammed into the room: some from the emergency department, and some from the ICU. They informed us that both units were full. So, I thought to myself, *what were we to do with this patient now?*

At this point in the transport, we had been at the hospital for about an hour. The charge nurse from the intensive care unit said they could move one patient but it would take about 45 minutes to an hour before the room would be ready. We could not leave her on the regular floor with a breathing tube in, so I offered to watch her until the room was ready. As I continued to breathe for the patient, I realized I had told the pilots we would be right back. One of my partners went back to the aircraft to inform them of the situation and get our portable ventilator to avoid needing to breathe for her manually. Minutes later, he came back with the ventilator and said we had a problem.

The pilots told him if we did not leave within an hour, they would duty time out and be forced to leave without us. Pilots are required by law to have the aircraft on the ground

14 hours after their shift begins. If they did not fly the aircraft back to base, the next crew would need to drive to the hospital and then fly it home.

Not knowing what to do, and having never encountered this situation before, I informed the charge nurse of the situation. The last thing I wanted was to arrange alternate transportation back to our base. Nevertheless, I told the charge nurse I'd wait as long as necessary for the bed to become available. The charge nurse said she would try to speed up things and I told her thank you. While waiting, I connected our patient to the transport ventilator to free up my hands. But just when I thought the transport couldn't get worse, it did.

The blood pressure cuff cycled and did not get a pressure. After placing the breathing tube, we had been taking a blood pressure every five minutes and using a finger probe to monitor oxygen levels. Now, neither displayed a reading. Our monitor showed she had electrical activity in her heart, but it was not pumping strong enough to get a blood pressure. We felt for a pulse in several locations, but it had vanished. We double checked, but it still was not there. I thought to myself that *placing a breathing tube if she did not want one was bad enough, but now we needed to start CPR*. We rechecked pulses. The doctor checked. The pulse still was not there and something had to be done or she would die. Still with no official code status, I said "we have to start CPR" and began doing chest compressions. We had no other choice. There was no documentation and nobody truly knew the patient's wishes. We did CPR for several minutes, and after a giving a few medications, our patient regained a pulse.

About 5 minutes later, the family made it to the hospital. They walked into the room in tears as they watched the ventilator breathing for their mother. Nobody talked, and the only sounds that could be heard came from the ventilator and her daughter weeping. Once her daughter regained composure, she whispered in a gentle, soft voice, "Mom would not want this," and began to cry again.

The physician took her outside the room and they spoke for several minutes. The family had known their mother didn't want a breathing tube, or CPR, but did not want to make that decision for her. They were hoping their mother would document all this after the hospital stay. Unfortunately, our patient could not communicate her wishes and we needed to know how to proceed, and what to do, from this point. The daughter called other family members and said that once the rest of the family arrived, they wanted to remove the breathing tube.

If the intensive care bed was not ready in 30 minutes, the pilots would have to leave without us. Although I wanted to get off work at a decent hour, it would have been heartless to pressure the hospital staff to hurry. I cannot imagine the emotional stress the family must have been experiencing. They were grieving, so I offered to stay as long as needed. Fifteen minutes later the bed was ready and we took the patient to the ICU. Nurses placed her on their monitoring equipment and the respiratory therapist connected her to the hospital ventilator. The charge nurse thanked us for being so patient and we hurried to get back to the aircraft, just in time to catch a flight back home.

The Outcome:

The patient had multiple strokes in her brain and never fully recovered. After discussions with family, an official do not resuscitate (DNR) order was placed in her medical record. The next morning, with the family at her bedside, hospital staff removed the breathing tube. After the tube was out, she did not expire, but she suffered significant neurological damage, and was then transferred from the hospital to a long-term care facility. She transferred back in and out of the hospital several times for various complications and was never herself again. I sometimes wonder what might have happened if I never started CPR, and I ask myself if I did the right thing.

Take Home Points:

For the Nurse or EMS Provider:

EMS – This is an ethical dilemma you might one day face. Even though we all want to respect patient's wishes, there can be legal consequences for withholding CPR. If you haven't thought about what you'd do if placed in this situation, I recommend you do so.

Nurses – Please make sure your patients have their wishes documented. If they don't, talk with them or their families about advanced directives and power of attorney. This can be a sensitive topic, but it's important to discuss these things ahead of time.

For the Public:

I shared this story to try and stress the importance of having BOTH an advanced health care directive AND a power of attorney. Do not force someone to make your health care decisions on your behalf. While beneficial to have someone to cover the medical choices you may not have thought of, imagine the stress of making these types of decisions for someone you love. Ask your doctor or a lawyer to help with this.

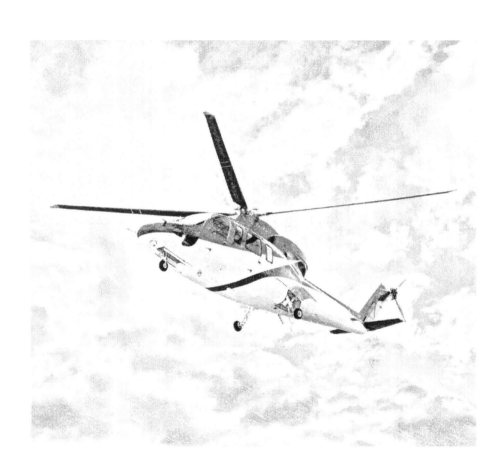

SEVERE PNEUMONIA

Setting:

A 68 year old man with a medical history of chronic obstructive pulmonary disease (COPD) and prior heart attacks, had been coughing for a week, and complained to his wife he was short of breath. This man despised visits to his doctor and had always been reluctant to seek medical advice. His wife, concerned for his safety, convinced him to get checked out by a local primary care physician. The physician thought his condition warranted admission to the small rural hospital down the street for closer observation and further testing. His wife drove him to this hospital and he was admitted to a bed on the regular nursing floor.

Once on the regular floor, the nurses agreed he was too sick for their unit. He began to sweat profusely and became anxious, which further worsened his breathing problem. The patient continued to deteriorate and the nursing staff called an emergency response team. This team consisted of three specialists, a critical care nurse from the intensive care unit, a respiratory therapist, and the single emergency department doc at the hospital. The team arrived minutes later and placed him on a 100% oxygen mask, called a non-rebreather. This improved his breathing slightly. They arranged for a bed on the intensive care unit for closer monitoring.

The physician in charge of the intensive care unit ordered several basic tests, but no definite cause of his condition could be found. He believed the patient had either pneumonia or fluid accumulation in his lungs. Since the hospital had limited resources to manage critically ill patients, it became clear to the physician and staff that this patient needed to be transferred to a higher level of care. The intensive care doctor made arrangements for transfer and requested helicopter for transport.

Everyday Language Of What Might Be Going On:

Several medical conditions can lead to difficulty breathing. Regardless of the underlying cause, tissues in the body do not get enough oxygen, triggering the sensation of shortness of breath. Often, one of the following processes might be occurring:

- Oxygen might not be getting into the blood from the lungs, as in pneumonia, pulmonary embolism, pulmonary edema, or COPD.
- The heart may not be pumping oxygen in the blood to the body's tissues, such as during a heart attack, atrial fibrillation, or other arrhythmia.
- The body may not have enough blood cells to carry oxygen to the tissues, as in anemia.
- The body may consume more oxygen than normal as in hyperthyroid or sepsis.
- Something might change the direction of blood flow to the tissues, such as heart valve problems or an aortic dissection.

Although many other potential causes for difficult breathing exist, these are conditions a doctor will want to rule out. Physicians use a collaboration of symptoms to help guide testing and make the proper diagnosis.

For example, with pulmonary edema or severe pneumonia, oxygen cannot get from the lungs to the blood. In pneumonia, bacterial or viral growth causes inflammation and fluid accumulation in air spaces (alveoli) of the lungs. Pulmonary edema is often caused by congestive heart failure from increased pulmonary vascular pressures. These higher pressures cause fluid to leak into the alveoli. This fluid blocks gas exchange, preventing oxygen from getting to the blood from the lungs.

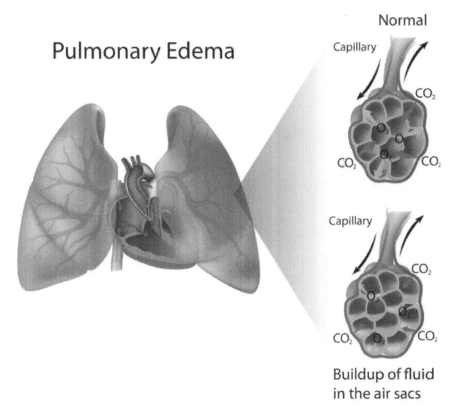

Pulmonary Edema

Normal

Capillary

CO_2

CO_2 CO_2

Capillary

CO_2

CO_2 CO_2

Buildup of fluid
in the air sacs

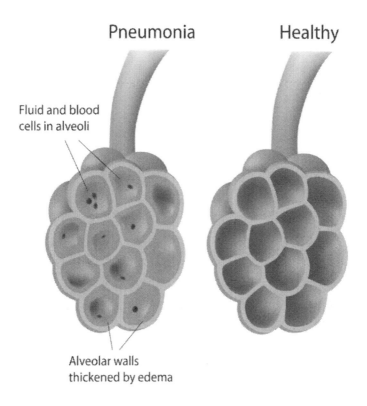

Pneumonia   Healthy

Fluid and blood
cells in alveoli

Alveolar walls
thickened by edema

For smokers, each time the smoke reaches the lungs it triggers a reaction, resulting in microscopic deposits of scar tissue. In turn, this scar tissue will not allow oxygen to pass through the lungs. The more a person smokes, the greater amount of scarring that forms in the lungs, and the more trouble he or she will have breathing. Other urgent diseases that need to be ruled out quickly for anyone with difficulty breathing include heart attack, heart rate problems, congestive heart failure or other heart problems, aortic dissection, collapsed lung, pneumonia, asthma attack, COPD exacerbation, pulmonary embolism, and anaphylactic shock.

There are several ways to help a person who is having trouble breathing. Which method works best depends on the underlying condition. The air we breathe contains roughly 21% oxygen and 78% nitrogen. One method often used to initially help with shortness of breath is to increase the percentage of oxygen a person breathes. This can be done with devices such as a nasal cannula, face mask, BiPAP (Bi-level Positive Airway Pressure) or CPAP (Continuous Positive Airway Pressure), and by placing a breathing tube.

A nasal cannula is a small plastic tube with nasal prongs. One end connects directly to a 100% oxygen source and the two prongs on the other end rest in the nose. The nasal cavity then fills with 100% oxygen at a selected rate of 1 to 6 liters per minute. But, the volume of gas a person breathes is larger than the nasal cavity. With each breath, the 100% oxygen in the nasal cavity mixes with 21% atmospheric oxygen to deliver roughly 24% to 44% oxygen to the lungs. The higher the selected oxygen flow rate, the greater percentage of oxygen delivered.

If the patient still requires more oxygen, a mask can be used to increase the percentage of oxygen that reaches the lungs. The mask acts as a larger reservoir than the nose for the 100% oxygen. When the patient breathes, a larger volume of 100% oxygen mixes with atmospheric oxygen, thus increasing the total percentage of oxygen delivered to the lungs.

To maximize the reservoir of oxygen, a bag can be connected to a face mask. This mask with a bag is called a non-rebreather. BiPAP and CPAP help a person by applying positive airway pressure to the lungs in addition to increasing the percentage of oxygen. When the above fail, a small plastic breathing tube can be placed through the mouth and into the trachea (windpipe). This tube can then be connected to a high pressure oxygen source and deliver 21% to 100% oxygen to the lungs at controlled volumes, rates, and pressures.

Oxygen Delivery Devices

Nasal Cannula

Oxygen Mask

Non-Rebreather

BiPAP / CPAP Mask

Ambu Bag Valve Mask

Endotracheal Tube

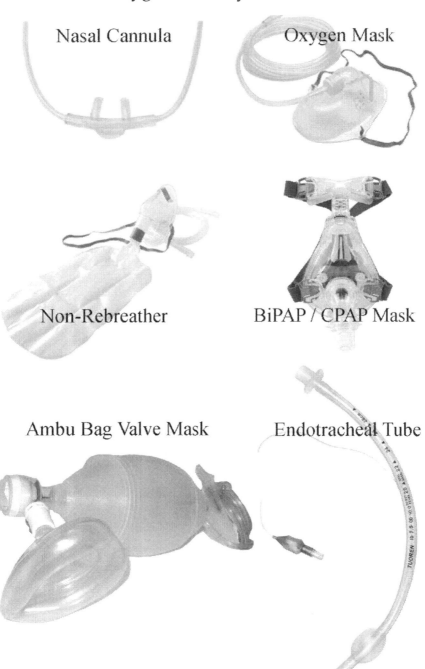

The Flight Out and Game Plan:

Our team was dispatched to a small rural hospital 90 miles away, a 25 to 30 minute helicopter flight. The only information relayed to us was our patient complained of shortness of breath, required a non-rebreathing mask with 100% oxygen, and had a history of COPD and prior heart attacks. Many things can cause shortness of breath, but based on his history, four potential causes came to mind: COPD exacerbation, severe pneumonia, congestive heart failure, or heart attack.

When a patient becomes acutely short of breath, they are often placed on 100% oxygen when they may not need that much. Clinicians administer oxygen at high levels attempting to quickly fix the problem then gradually lower the amount. But, if patients have trouble breathing with 100% oxygen, the situation is critical. BiPAP or CPAP are modes of ventilation that might improve certain conditions. However, if the patient cannot breathe on a 100% non-rebreathing oxygen mask, the next step in management is often to place a breathing tube. I wanted to know if the 100% non-rebreather improved our patients breathing difficulties and if he truly needed that much. If his symptoms resolved after the mask had been applied, the transport would probably be straightforward. Unfortunately, this would prove to not be the case.

On the flight out, we radioed our dispatch center to ask for an update about the patient's status and requested his weight. Drugs used for intubation are dosed by weight and we wanted to calculate the doses ahead of time. If our patient needed a breathing tube, we wanted to be prepared. Dispatch telephoned the hospital and relayed back to us both his weight and a status update. He was getting worse, and weighed much more than we had expected at over 300 pounds. Although this made our calculations easy because he needed the max dose of any intubation drugs we planned to give him, it ensured a more difficult transport for several reasons.

Larger people are more difficult to move, tend to deteriorate faster, and it's usually more challenging to place a breathing tube in these patients. Ideally when placing a breathing tube, medications are given to both sedate and paralyze patients. Sedation takes away a person's normal drive to breathe and after giving a paralytic, they are no longer capable of breathing. Larger people tend to have less of an oxygen reserve, meaning their oxygen levels drop much faster than normal after giving these medications. Additionally, the excess tissue in their neck makes finding the correct anatomic location to place the tube more difficult. This combination makes placing a breathing tube in larger people more frightening and dangerous.

The Transport:

We landed ten minutes later and a security guard escorted us to the intensive care unit. I peeked into our patient's room and knew with first glance he was not doing well, but thought perhaps he might be stable enough to avoid intubation. The nurse gave us a brief report and we placed him on our transport monitor. He had a fast heart rate in the 130s and high blood pressure of 184/94. His oxygen saturation level was concerning, but still in the low normal range with a reading of 90%.

When I asked him how he felt on the 100% oxygen mask, he said he was doing better but it got worse whenever he moved. I talked with his doctor, who had been waiting for us at the hospital, but few clues pointed to a clear diagnosis. The physician thought this might be either a case of severe pneumonia or pulmonary edema with too much fluid in his lungs. But, because of the limited capabilities of the hospital, only a handful of tests had been done, none of which definitively diagnosed the problem.

His electrocardiogram did not indicate he was having an acute heart attack and he denied having any chest, arm, back, or abdominal pain. I listened to his heart and lung sounds with my stethoscope. His heart sounded normal but I heard an abnormality in both lower lung fields. This abnormality may well have been caused by his underlying COPD, by pneumonia, or by fluid in his lungs. His chest x-ray showed signs of either pneumonia or fluid, but which was it? We did not know, and would not know, until further testing could be done at the other hospital. Our goal was to keep him alive and oxygenating until these questions could be answered later.

The sending physician had given a medication, called a diuretic, to remove excess fluid from the patient's body. A foley catheter had also been placed to monitor his urine output. If it was fluid seen on the chest x-ray, the diuretic might help remove fluid from the lungs and improve his breathing. They gave aspirin in case it was a heart attack, as well as the first drugs commonly given for patients having a COPD exacerbation. Antibiotics had been ordered to treat a possible pneumonia, but had not yet been administered.

These treatments all seemed reasonable but might have taken too long to work. He needed something to help his breathing now. We started an intravenous (IV) infusion, called nitroglycerin, to both reduce his blood pressure and dilate the vascular system. This might help with all of the potential problems mentioned. It would lower his blood pressure, creating less work for the heart. Dilating the vasculature might allow a space for the fluid to accumulate other than in the lungs. If he was having a heart attack, this might increase blood flow to the heart. After 10 minutes at the bedside preparing for transport, we decided he was stable enough for the flight and lifted him to our transport cot. This, unfortunately, proved to be a turning point for the patient.

We placed him on the transport cot and his condition deteriorated. He was no longer stable enough for transfer. The minimal movement from the hospital bed to our cot had triggered his heart rate to increase from the 130s to the 150s. He said it was much more difficult to breathe, and his oxygen levels had plummeted to well below normal, now in the 80s. Something to improve his condition needed to be done before leaving the unit.

Since he was already on a 100% non-rebreather oxygen mask, we had two options that might help: put him on a different kind of breathing mask and connect it to a machine called BiPAP or CPAP, or place a breathing tube now. BiPAP and CPAP both apply continual pressure to the lungs and might redistribute the fluid from his lungs back into the vasculature, allowing for better gas exchange. Nobody knew for certain that fluid in his lungs was the problem, though, and it might not help for pneumonia. BiPAP and CPAP are both less dangerous than placing a breathing tube, but if they did not work, he would need to be intubated anyway. Since we had a rather long flight ahead of us, we decided to place the tube before leaving and not take any chances. Placing a breathing tube in the small confinements of a helicopter did not sound like the safest choice.

We asked the patient if we could place a breathing tube to help with his symptoms and he quickly agreed. Still on our cot, we put him in an optimal position for successful placement of the tube. He was overweight, with a large neck. This usually makes placing the tube more challenging, so we prepared our backup equipment in case we needed to resort to alternative airway measures. We decided to avoid the traditional intubation approach and placed the tube with a video-aided device called a glidescope.

My partner gave the patient a sedative and made sure we could ventilate him before giving a paralytic medication. The worst case scenario would be to have this guy paralyzed and not be able to place the tube or ventilate him. After he was adequately sedated, I removed the mask from his face and placed a different type of mask over his nose and mouth that connected to a device called an ambu bag. This device allowed us to manually breathe for him. During an intubation, the placement of the tube can sometimes cause vomiting. To prevent this, we give a medication that paralyzes the body. Once I knew I could ventilate him, my partner administered a paralytic so our patient would not aspirate stomach contents into his lungs. His condition was already critical and stomach contents in the lungs would only worsen the situation.

I felt my heart beat a bit faster as I lowered the head of the cot, positioning him for intubation. I removed the mask and placed the glidescope in his mouth, looked toward the video screen, and saw a beautiful picture...his pearly white vocal cords.

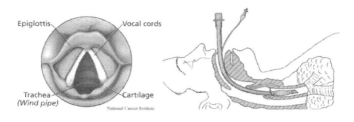

Epiglottis
Vocal cords
Trachea (Wind pipe)
Cartilage
National Cancer Institute

I manipulated the breathing tube through the cords and inflated a small balloon near the end of the tube. This balloon is around the plastic tube and inflates in the trachea, or windpipe, creating a seal that helps to prevent oral secretions from traveling into the lungs. I removed the mask from the ambu bag and then connected it to the breathing tube. We confirmed the tube was in the trachea, and not the esophagus, by listening for breath sounds over his lungs and measuring the carbon dioxide leaving the tube. His lungs would rise, and then gradually fall, with each breath I gave him. What a relief knowing the tube was in the right spot.

Several minutes later, he started to look much better and appeared more stable. His heart rate and blood pressure began to return to normal. His skin began to pink up and he looked like he was in a peaceful dream. We gathered our supplies, grabbed the antibiotic from the nurse, and left the hospital. Once we loaded him into the aircraft cabin, we connected our transport ventilator to the breathing tube. The sedative we had given began to wear off and he started to waken, so we kept him comfortable throughout the flight by giving him two more doses of sedation. We also administered the antibiotic the sending hospital had given us to treat his possible pneumonia. The rest of the transport to the accepting hospital was uneventful. We landed 30 minutes later and took him to his new intensive care bed for further testing, then flew back to base and made sure everything was in order for our next mission.

The Outcome:

He did end up having a severe pneumonia along with a minor heart attack. He also had an undiagnosed heart failure, which was only apparent after further testing. It's likely that because of his underlying heart failure and obesity, his body was unable to tolerate the pneumonia, contributing to his respiratory symptoms and small heart attack. He was extubated while completing a 10 day course of antibiotics, placed on heart failure medications, and discharged home. He was scheduled for a cardiac catheterization to determine if abnormalities to his coronary blood flow existed. Unfortunately, I was unable to find the results of the catheterization or determine if he ever had it.

Take Home Points:

For the Nurse or EMS Provider:

Nitroglycerin (NTG) helps reduce preload and afterload. In patients with congestive heart failure, NTG is often one of the first drugs ordered. By dilating the venous system the drug provides a space for intravascular fluid to accumulate other than the lungs. By reducing afterload, it allows the heart to increase output and helps get the diuretic to the kidney. In addition, it may help dilate coronary arteries and increase blood flow to the heart.

BiPAP and CPAP are used for patients in congestive heart failure who present with signs of fluid overload - the positive pressure applied to the lungs will help push excess fluid into the pulmonary vasculature and prevent further fluid from accumulating in the lungs.

Realize that we will never be experts in intubation and always prepare before starting this procedure.

- While you get everything ready, make sure the patient is on 100% oxygen. If he is already on BiPAP...turn the FiO_2 up to 100%.
- Equipment –line with pressure applied in case you need to give fluid rapidly and for pushing medications, suction, ambu bag, mask, oxygen at 15 liters, laryngoscope and blades, ETT and a size smaller (7.5 is a good choice for the average size adult), stylet, syringe to inflate the cuff, $ETCO_2$ confirmation, drugs ready to go, anticipate depth of tube (24cm normal man, 22cm normal woman), stethoscope.

- Have several backup plans and equipment ready: laryngeal mask airway, bougie, glidescope, surgical airway, etc.
- Assess your ability to ventilate before pushing a paralytic because once you push that paralytic; you will be in full control of ventilation.

For the Public:

Young and healthy people can handle pneumonia easier than the elderly and those with other diseases. If you're older or have other medical problems, do not take a cough lightly. Bacteria growing in your lungs can block the exchange of gas which only worsens as the bacteria spread throughout the lungs. Get treatment for difficulty breathing early.

Patients with heart failure may experience shortness of breath because of excess fluid accumulation in the lungs. A weak heart cannot keep up with excessive fluid in the vasculature. If you notice ankle swelling, weight gain, shortness of breath, difficulty lying flat, fatigue, persistent coughing or wheezing (especially if white or pink tinged mucus). Get it checked out.

JEHOVAH'S WITNESS AORTIC DISSECTION

Setting:

A 52-year-old Jehovah's Witness male with a medical history of hypertension had just gotten home from a Sunday religious service when he felt a sudden, excruciating, and tearing chest pain. Concerned about a heart attack, his wife called 911, and an ambulance arrived within minutes. He still complained of a terrible chest pain. The paramedics gave him 4 baby aspirin, put the man on their monitor, lifted him to the cot, and loaded him into the ambulance. They then drove to the nearest hospital, which happened to be the major trauma center of this metropolitan city.

At the emergency room, his chest pain had not improved so he was given the narcotic morphine. The attending physician asked the man several questions about his past medical history. Apparently, his hypertension had been difficult to control in the past, and several of his relatives had been diagnosed with aortic aneurysms. The physician performed a physical examination and discovered one of the man's radial pulses, which are the pulses in his wrist, felt stronger than the other. His heart rate ranged higher than normal at 100 to 105 beats per minute and blood pressures taken in both arms confirmed a difference in pulse strength. The blood pressure was 185/90 in the right arm and 155/80 in the left arm. Pulses in his right foot were gone and could barely be felt in the left.

Imaging confirmed the diagnosis of aortic dissection; this was one of the most extensive dissections this doctor had ever heard of or seen. His aorta had a tear from its beginning just past the heart, up the ascending aorta, across the arch, and all the way down to the mid-thigh. Blood work was sent and a surgeon consulted to see if the problem might be repairable. The blood results suggested that he was slowly bleeding internally. If his dissection was not repaired in the next several hours, he would have no chance of survival. Unfortunately, the surgeon at that hospital was not willing to operate unless the patient agreed to accept blood products.

The patient, steadfast to his faith, refused to receive them, even in the face of imminent death. The emergency department physician made several phone calls to the largest medical centers in the state and surrounding states. He found one center willing to evaluate the patient, but they would not guarantee a surgical attempt at repair if the patient continued to refuse blood products. The medical center that accepted the patient for evaluation was almost 200 miles from this emergency department. With no other options, the physician initiated transfer and requested a helicopter for rapid air medical transport.

Everyday Language Of What Might Be Going On:

The aorta has three layers: an inner lining, middle layer, and an outer layer. In an aortic dissection, the inner lining tears and blood travels through this tear, dissecting the inner and/or middle layer from the outer. Dissections involving the aortic arch, as in this case, are a surgical emergency and must be corrected as soon as possible. If the outer layer ruptures, rapid blood loss ensues, and most patients will die before any attempt can be made to fix it.

This patient had several risk factors for aortic dissection, including a history of uncontrolled hypertension and a family history of aortic aneurysm. Aortic dissection pain is often described as a tearing, or ripping, pain across the chest and/or back between the shoulder blades. This pain may extend to other areas of the body, such as the lower back or abdomen, as the dissection expands. However, pain or exam abnormalities are not always present in patients with aortic dissection.

If the dissection involves the hearts aortic valve, an abnormal heart sound called a murmur is sometimes heard. Blood pressures can be higher on different sides of the body because of the tear and abnormalities of blood flow. Pulse differences in the arms or legs suggest dissection as noted in this case. If blood flow from organs is obstructed because of the dissection, organs might not function properly and further pain may occur in those areas. Our patient had a tearing pain, family history, unequal pulses, and a murmur sometimes caused by aortic dissection.

Healthcare professionals must differentiate a heart attack from aortic dissection as fast as possible. Immediate treatment for a heart attack involves administration of drugs to prevent clotting. Conversely, clotting abnormalities in aortic dissection are corrected as soon as possible. Improper treatment can cause devastating consequences. Once dissection is suspected, the confirmatory test is usually a computed tomography (CT) scan which shows two distinct channels of blood when only one should be seen. After aortic dissection is confirmed and surgical repair deemed necessary, treatment is focused on lowering the heart rate and blood pressure, correcting bleeding abnormalities, and preparing for emergent surgical repair.

This patient had a high risk for major complications including death. His dissection was huge and he would almost certainly need multiple blood products with any surgical attempt at repair. To further complicate his problem, he had received aspirin by the paramedics who gave this because they attributed his chest pain to a heart attack. Aspirin alters platelet function and delays blood clotting time, making those who take it more prone to bleeding. Jehovah's Witnesses are not allowed to receive whole blood, or any of its components (red cells, white cells, platelets, or plasma). Even if he went to surgery, his chances of survival remained extremely poor.

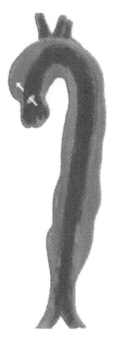

The Flight Out and Game Plan:

Early into a night shift, we had just finished our evening briefing and, as I poured a cup of coffee, my pager vibrated. I read the text and did not believe what I read…."52-year-old male, Jehovah Witness, Type A dissection, H/H 10/30, sending surgeon will not operate". H/H is an abbreviation for hemoglobin and hematocrit which are measurements of blood volume. The normal hemoglobin for most males ranges from 14 to 17. His was 10. It looked as if his aorta might be leaking. The pilots accepted the flight and we were airborne minutes later.

Several factors of this transport concerned me. First, the patient had received aspirin which might alter his natural ability to stop any bleeding. More importantly though, because of his religious belief, if he had any bleeding problems or his blood pressure dropped, we could not give blood products to correct these issues. These might be the difference between our patient arriving to the operating room alive or dead.

When a person is actively bleeding, it's usually preferred to replace the lost blood with blood and/or blood products. Sometimes intravenous (IV) fluids might help, but they aren't as effective. This patient needed to be in the operating room an hour ago. I was worried that in the 30 minutes it took us to get there, or the hour flight to the accepting hospital, the dissection might rupture. If it ruptured before arriving at the accepting hospital he probably would not survive the transport. Even if we made it to the accepting hospital, the surgeon still had to agree to perform surgery, and our patient had to survive the surgery without blood. The chances of a good outcome were extremely small. But, you never know which transports will be one of those "miracle patients," so you treat each of them with the expectation that they'll go home.

The Transport:

If this man had any chance to live, time was critical to his survival. As luck would have it, or shall I say not have it, the pilots could not land the helicopter on this helipad because of construction issues. This forced us to land at an alternate landing zone located a few miles away and take an ambulance to the hospital, further delaying the transport. We landed, unloaded our cot and equipment, and loaded it into the awaiting ambulance. The driver of the squad made great time. He drove like a race car driver and we arrived at the hospital in less than 5 minutes.

This particular emergency department had a reputation for being one of the best trauma centers in the state. Usually patients are flown into, not out of there. Security escorted us through several smaller subdivisions of the main emergency department until we came to our patient's room. The attending physician had just finished placing an arterial line. This allowed us to continually monitor our patients' blood pressure during the transport.

The physician gave us a brief report, but we already understood the severity of the situation and need for rapid transport. Many of the transports we do require us to place added intravenous lines to have adequate IV access but this emergency room had it done for us. You could tell it was a top-notch center. They had prepared to promptly give IV fluid if needed and had placed several large IVs. We placed the patient on our monitor and connected two IV lines in case his blood pressure dropped and we needed to give IV fluid.

The patient's pain had improved after receiving the morphine, but fear was visible in both his and his wife's facial expressions. His wife asked if she could fly with us. Expecting these to be the last hours of this man's life and the only time they would ever spend together again, we said yes. We connected our monitoring equipment, put him on our cot, and then left the emergency department.

I asked the ambulance driver to drive fast yet as smooth as possible, afraid that excessive shaking and moving might cause the dissection to rupture. Treatment goals for an aortic dissection are to reduce the shearing stress in the aorta. We attempt this by giving medications to first lower the heart rate to around 60 and then lower the systolic blood pressure (top number) near 100 and below 120. Our goal is to keep the pressure as low as possible yet still provide organs with adequate blood flow. By this time, however, his systolic blood pressure was already around 100 with no medical intervention except the morphine he had received for pain. Although his blood pressure was at goal, his heart rate was in the mid-90s, and slowing this further might lower his blood pressure too much. This combination of symptoms suggested to us that his intravascular volume was gradually depleting and his aorta, the main blood vessel in the body, was leaking.

Once at the helicopter, we unloaded the patient from the ambulance, then loaded and secured him in the aircraft cabin. His wife sat with us in the back. We secured her in her seat and put hearing protection on them both. The pilots went through their start-up checks while we positioned our equipment in the cabin. We placed the IV bags into pressurized devices, called pressure bags, which would increase the rate of fluid flowing into his veins once we opened the IV line. If he needed fluid, we wanted to be prepared to give it right away. After everything was secured, the pilots asked if we were ready and we lifted for the hour flight to the accepting hospital.

Twenty minutes into the flight, his heart rate increased to the 100s and his blood pressure trended down to 90/42. His heart rate increased to maintain normal blood flow as his internal volume depleted and his blood pressure decreased. With a systolic pressure below 90, further complications might develop. He was leaking internally and each minute that went by lowered his chances of survival. He needed IV fluid, but too much might contribute to further bleeding. I opened the IV line, giving just enough fluid to get his systolic pressure above 100, and then stopped it. Things looked decent for a while, but 15 minutes later the scenario repeated, and we again opened the IV fluid until his systolic blood pressure reached 100. He continued to slowly bleed out in front of us. This happened one more time, 5 minutes before landing, and we repeated the process.

Once on the ground at our destination, a sense of relief came over me. *Almost there,* I said to myself. The pilots powered-off the aircraft and we unloaded the patient as his wife watched. We took him to the intensive care unit as the wife followed and were greeted by several surgeons who had been waiting our arrival. They knew the urgency of the situation and wanted to waste no time evaluating him. We gave them the imaging disks the hospital had sent with us and they began to load the CT scans in the computer. My partner and I then helped the nurses place our patient in his assigned bed and hook him up to their monitoring equipment.

I walked out of the room and asked the surgeons what they thought. They still weren't sure if they would take him to the operating room and said that even if the patient accepted blood he probably would not survive the surgery. It was a strange sensation to watch our patient talking with his wife. Their facial expressions showed their deep sorrow and fear. The odds were not in his favor and those words they shared in that conversation may have been their last. I went back in the room, wished the family the best and walked out silently, grateful for my family's health, wondering what I would say to my wife and children if I were in his shoes.

The Outcome:

A month after this flight, I transported another patient to the very hospital unit where this man had been transferred. As I finished with the new patient, the former patient's wife came to greet me and updated me on his progress. The surgeons elected to give him a chance and took him to the operating room within an hour of his arrival. They emphasized that, without blood, he would likely not survive the surgery but without surgical intervention, he would surely die.

Jehovah's Witnesses can accept their own blood, but only if taken during the procedure: they cannot donate ahead of time. Technology which recycles lost blood was utilized during the procedure. He survived the surgery, but came out with extremely low blood levels, which may have contributed to later kidney injury for which he needed several weeks of dialysis. Measures were taken to avoid drawing too much blood for lab testing, his levels eventually improved, and his kidneys recovered. He left the hospital 2 months later. This was a true miracle story.

For the Nurse or EMS Provider:

Stanford Type A dissections include any dissection of the ascending aorta. They can have involvement with or without the arch and descending aorta.

Stanford Type B dissections do not include the ascending aorta. These are dissections that involve the descending thoracic aorta, which begins distal to the left subclavian artery, and/or the abdominal aorta.

Initial management of both type A and B dissections involves lowering the heart rate with IV beta blockade first. Once the heart rate has been lowered to around 60 bpm, if blood pressure is still above 110-120 mmHg systolic, vasodilators are then added for a goal of 100-120 mmHg[1].

Aortic Dissection
Type A   Type B

For the Public:

Hypertension can contribute to a multitude of health problems, including increasing your risk for aortic dissection, and it's important to get it under control.

Aortic dissection is somewhat uncommon and most frequently occurs in men between 60 and 70 years of age, although anyone can have it.

Symptoms may be like those of other heart issues, such as a heart attack.

The most common signs are: sudden severe chest or upper back pain, often described as a tearing, ripping or shearing sensation, that radiates to the neck or down the back.

Other potential symptoms include a loss of consciousness, shortness of breath, weakness, stroke like symptoms, and sweating or varying pulse pressures in the arms.

V-FIB CARDIAC ARREST

Setting:

A 59-year-old man was home vacuuming when he suddenly collapsed. His wife heard a loud thump and rushed to see what had created the noise. She ran into the living room and spotted her husband lying unconscious on the floor. In shock and not knowing what to do, she immediately called 911. The operator advised her to check for a pulse but she could not find one. The operator told her to start cardiopulmonary resuscitation (CPR) and continue until help arrived.

Paramedics came within minutes, found the wife doing chest compressions and took over CPR. They placed him on a monitor and his electrocardiograph (ECG) heart rhythm showed ventricular fibrillation (V-fib) cardiac arrest. His heart quivered in a lethal rhythm and if not corrected within minutes, the patient would die. The medics placed electrical defibrillation pads over his heart and shocked him into a normal heart rhythm. Once in a normal rhythm, his pulses returned but he remained unresponsive. They placed a breathing tube and took him to the closest emergency department located 5 minutes away. The patient began seizing while en route, violently shaking his body in the back of the ambulance.

Upon arrival to the hospital, he continued to seize and was given the drug lorazepam. It took some time for the medication to take effect but the seizure stopped several minutes later. The emergency department staff stabilized the patient, but this hospital could not offer the most current treatments available to optimize his chances at a full recovery. This man required percutaneous coronary intervention (PCI) to determine if an obstruction in coronary blood flow triggered the arrhythmia, and hypothermic cooling for 24 hours to minimize neurologic damage. The physician initiated transfer to the closest hospital capable of PCI and cooling measures, and requested a helicopter for rapid transport.

Everyday Language Of What Might Be Going On:

In a normal heart beat, each beat is generated from a location known as the sinoatrial node, or SA node. When the beat originates from the SA node, an electrical impulse travels in a distinct pattern, which allows the heart to beat at an optimal level. If electrical impulses arise from other areas of the heart, the heart's ability to effectively pump blood is compromised.

Ventricular fibrillation (V-fib) is an arrhythmia in which the heart has no output. A patient in ventricular fibrillation usually collapses within seconds from lack of blood flow to the brain. If not treated promptly, the patient can stop breathing and/or the pulse can completely stop. In V-fib, electrical impulses originate from multiple areas of the heart ventricles, resulting in a quivering heart. A patient in V-fib is defibrillated with the hope that each of these impulses will be stopped simultaneously and the SA node will again pace the heart. Once the SA node again becomes the core electrical impulse, the heart will begin to beat normally. The sooner a person in V-fib is defibrillated, the more likely the arrhythmia can be restored to a normal rhythm. The main goal of CPR is to perfuse vital organs until a normal or perfusing rhythm can be restored.

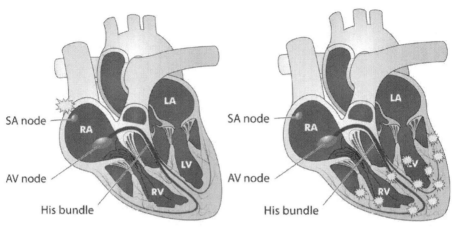

Normal - Sinoatrial Node   Ventricular Fibrillation

Ventricular fibrillation is most commonly linked to ongoing heart attacks or prior scarring of the heart muscle from a previous heart attack. Once the patient has been stabilized after V-fib arrest, it's important to find the cause of the arrhythmia. In certain situations, patients are cooled as soon as possible after the cardiac arrest to improve outcomes. The patient may need cardiac catheterization to examine coronary blood flow. If flow abnormalities are found, he/she may need stenting or coronary artery bypass grafting. If they recover, they may need to take medications to prevent future arrhythmias and preserve cardiac function. They may also have an internal defibrillator placed to correct life threatening arrhythmias before the patient becomes symptomatic, or have an ablation of abnormal electrical pathways.

The Flight Out and Game Plan:

Our team was dispatched to a small rural hospital 45 miles away from our base, approximately a 15 minute flight. We walked to the aircraft and were airborne in minutes. A medical student with aspirations of becoming an emergency room physician happened to be flying with us that day. Sometimes, observers can slow the transport, but having an extra set of hands proved beneficial on this flight.

We knew the patient had been in V-fib cardiac arrest but now was reported to be somewhat stable with a pulse and perfusing rhythm. This still concerned us because it's fairly common for patients to go back in to V-fib, or have other potentially fatal arrhythmias, after having been in V-fib. The sending and accepting physicians thought poor blood flow to the heart (coronary ischemia) caused the episode of V-fib arrest. Our dispatch center instructed us to take him directly to the cardiac catheterization lab, where they would try to open the obstructing vessel.

The plan was for me to put the patient on our monitor and place defibrillation pads before I did anything else. If he did go into an arrhythmia, we wanted to be able to shock his heart into a normal rhythm as fast as possible. While I did this, my partner would hurry to place an arterial line. In transport, because of constant movements and vibrations, we sometimes see what is known as "artifact" on our monitor.

Artifact is the appearance of an abnormal heart rhythm, such as V-fib, when no abnormality or arrhythmia is truly present. If he did go back into V-fib, we might mistake this initially for artifact and take longer to identify and correct it. The arterial line would allow us to monitor his blood pressure continuously with each heartbeat, every second of the transport. With an acute drop in blood pressure, we could then instantly differentiate a potentially fatal arrhythmia from artifact. We wanted to be fast at the bedside and get him somewhere more capable of handling this condition, so we planned to manually bag and breathe for the patient instead of taking extra time to set up the ventilator.

The Transport:

The helipad at this particular hospital was almost a half mile from the emergency department (ED), so an ambulance had been arranged to drive us to the ED. We landed near the hospital, the pilots powered-off the aircraft, and we loaded our cot and equipment into the ambulance which drove us to the ED. The medical team on the ambulance, coincidently, was the same crew who responded to the 911 call. They told us their version of what had happened and offered their help. We asked how the patient was doing and they responded, "Not too good."

During the minute drive, I looked over toward the medical student, who had a blank stare on his face. I whispered to him, "this should be exciting", and he offered to help. Uncertain about his qualifications, I thanked him but asked if he could stand and observe from a distance. He said "okay" and before I knew it, the ambulance stopped, we unloaded our equipment, and we entered our patient's room.

On the hospital gurney lay a lifeless man with a breathing tube in his mouth. The room was silent, almost tranquil. The only whisper or movements came from each ventilator breath as air moved in and out of his lungs. He seemed rather stable, considering the fact CPR had been performed on him less than an hour earlier. His heart rhythm, blood pressure, and oxygen status were all normal... at least for the time being anyway. I could sense the tension from the hospital staff. Everyone knew that at any instant, his heart might go back into V-fib.

The physician and nurses quickly gave us the story and said he had just stopped seizing several minutes before we got there. Two intravenous (IV) infusions were running; one called heparin, the other lidocaine. If this was a heart attack, heparin might prevent further obstruction in coronary blood vessels. Lidocaine had been started to help prevent another episode of V-fib. Unfortunately, lidocaine can potentially induce seizures and there was no guarantee the lidocaine would prevent V-fib from happening again. We quickly went to work, hoping neither would occur.

I placed him on our monitor and put defibrillation pads over his heart while my partner set up to place an arterial line. These pads stuck to his body and then connected to our monitor. If he needed shocked, we would be able to do this in a matter of seconds. Once he was on our monitor I moved to the IV infusions. This hospital had the same IV tubing we used, which made the transition quicker. Although lidocaine could potentially induce another seizure, we chose to keep it going to prevent another episode of ventricular fibrillation. By the time I finished placing both IV infusions on our pumps, my partner had placed the arterial line and we connected it to our monitor. Now we could see his blood pressure every time his heart contracted.

His vital signs still appeared stable and, with the help of the paramedics and pilots, we put him on our transport cot. Next, we removed the patient from the hospital ventilator and applied our end tidal carbon dioxide (ETCO$_2$) monitor. This measures the amount of carbon dioxide leaving the patient through the breathing tube to better gauge his ventilation status. Ten minutes after arriving, we left the bedside, manually breathing for our patient with an ambu bag. I thought to myself, *that went pretty smooth*, but I had just jinxed myself.

Seconds after loading our patient into the ambulance, I noticed a life-threatening arrhythmia on our monitor. It wasn't V-fib, but this rhythm can be just as dangerous and often progresses to V-fib. He had gone into ventricular tachycardia (V-tach.) with a heart rate in the 190s.

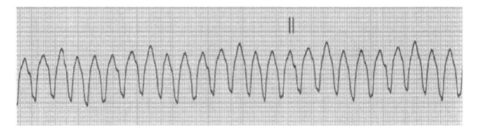

His heart beat so fast there was barely enough time for it to fill with blood. The heart pumped, but little blood flowed out of it. The arterial line tracing verified this was real because his blood pressure had plummeted.

We had to get him out of this rhythm or he would die. I yelled "we have to shock him." There were several of us in the back of the ambulance: a pilot and co-pilot, a medical student, one paramedic, my partner, and myself. None of us wanted to get shocked. I charged our monitor to the maximal defibrillating power and yelled "clear," made sure no one was touching our patient or the cot, and defibrillated him.

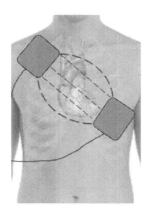

What seemed like minutes, but was in fact only seconds after the defibrillation, he had returned to his normal rhythm. We had to prevent this from occurring again and my partner said to give him another dose of lidocaine. He had this IV infusion running but now needed a large bolus dose. Since I had been manually breathing for our patient, I needed to free up my hands to get the medication from our bag. I asked the medical student if he wanted to learn how to use an ambu bag to breathe for a patient. He looked somewhat stunned but said sure. I showed him how to use the ambu bag and told him to squeeze every 4 or 5 seconds and we would tell him if he needed to speed up or slow down his rate. The medical student took over breathing for our patient and I grabbed the lidocaine out of our bag. By this time we had arrived at the helicopter and I gave the lidocaine. We unloaded the patient from the ambulance and started to load him into the helicopter.

Halfway into the aircraft cabin, the patient began to forcefully move his right arm, perhaps having another seizure, and I noticed blood on his forearm. One of his IVs had come out and we needed to start another one before we did anything else. His only IV already had an infusion running through it. If he went into another arrhythmia, we would not have enough IV access to treat it. The only place to put one, though, was on the shaking arm. His other arm already had an IV and an arterial line. The pilot held his arm still while I placed and secured another IV. We gave a medication called lorazepam (Ativan) to stop his seizure and further sedate him to keep him from moving. Minutes later, the arm shaking faded as we finished loading him into the aircraft.

The pilots began starting the helicopter while we secured everything in the cabin, continually monitoring our patient. We lifted and began the 15 minute flight to the accepting hospital with one eye glued to the monitor and the other on the patient. Fortunately, the flight was quick and our patient remained stable. There were no more serious arrhythmias or arm shaking, and he stayed still for the flight. The medical student continued to breathe for the patient for the rest of the transport. Even though we no longer needed his help, he was doing a good job and wanted the learning experience. We landed, unloaded the patient, and took him to the cardiac catheterization lab where a team was waiting our arrival. We put him on the cath lab table and the cath team began their attempt and saving this patient.

The Outcome:

The patient had a coronary angiogram and a stent placed followed by hypothermic cooling for 24 hours. He had a full neurological recovery and went home within two weeks. About two months after the flight, this kind gentleman surprised me with the best banana cream pie I had ever eaten and we talked about what happened that day. He thanked me over and over, but if his wife and paramedics had not provided quality CPR and early defibrillation, the outcome would not have been the same.

Take Home Points:

For the Nurse or EMS Provider:

Although many factors contributed to this great outcome, it's the EMS providers in the field who responded to the call that gave this man a second chance at life. They performed quality CPR, defibrillated immediately, and brought this man back to life.

For the Public:

Take a class and learn CPR: you might save the life of someone you love. Had the wife not started CPR at once, he would have had little chance for survival. High-quality CPR, especially good and effective chest compressions, contributes significantly to the successful resuscitation of patients with cardiac arrest.

CPR should be performed until professionals arrive and generally is:

- 30 chest compressions to the heart and then two resuscitation breaths (goal is 100-120 compressions per minute)
- Many health care professionals now say that mouth to mouth breathing may not be necessary and just compressions are sufficient.

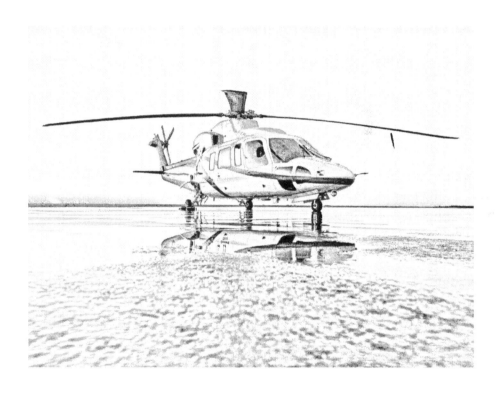

SUBARACHNOID HEMORRHAGE AFTER SEX

Setting:

A 32 year old man experienced a 4 second loss of consciousness while having sex with his girlfriend. They had been up most of the night partying, smoking marijuana, and drinking alcohol before the event. After passing out, he felt a terrible headache and became nauseous. He got up from bed, took two Percocet, and then lay back down with his girlfriend, who noticed he was not quite his normal self and seemed excessively drowsy. Not sure what was going on, the girlfriend called 911.

An ambulance arrived several minutes later and the man appeared to be intoxicated. Paramedics smelled alcohol on his breath and asked the girlfriend if the two had been drinking or using any illicit drugs. She said "yes...but only marijuana and beer, nothing else...we've smoked before and he never acts like this." The man seemed confused and reluctant to leave, but the paramedics convinced him to go to the hospital. During the short drive, they started an intravenous (IV) line and gave a drug called Narcan, suspecting his symptoms might be from a narcotic overdose. Narcan is a drug used to reverse the effects of narcotics and might reverse the effects of Percocet, but would do nothing for the alcohol or marijuana. After the paramedics gave the Narcan, nothing improved and his symptoms did not change.

The ambulance arrived at the emergency department (ED) about 10 minutes later, at around 1 o'clock in the morning, with the patient still drowsy and confused. Once at the ED, his urine tested positive for both marijuana and opiates. Blood tests showed an alcohol level of more than double the legal intoxication limit. Narcan had already been given to reverse the effects of the Percocet, but no drug can reverse the effects of alcohol and marijuana. The physician and nursing staff attributed the confusion and drowsiness to alcohol and marijuana and decided to let him sleep it off at the hospital.

When the next shift came in the following morning, the patient had not improved and the oncoming physician ordered a computed tomography (CT) scan of the head to rule out a stroke. The CT showed a major subarachnoid hemorrhage. The patient did not get better because he had been bleeding into his brain. Since the hospital was not equipped to manage this condition, they called for helicopter transport to the closest neurosurgical stroke center.

Everyday Language Of What Might Be Going On:

The textbook complaint of a person presenting with subarachnoid hemorrhage (SAH) is 'they experience the worst headache of their life'. The brain is covered by several thin layers, and the subarachnoid space is an area between two of those layers. SAH is a type of intracranial bleed that results from a sudden escape of blood into the subarachnoid space, most often caused by a ruptured aneurysm. This is a life-threatening condition which must be treated at a center specialized to manage this condition. As blood flows out of the cerebral vasculature and into the cranial vault, the pressure increases and compresses brain tissue, resulting in headache, altered level of consciousness, restlessness, drowsiness, and agitation. SAH also lowers a persons threshold for having a seizure. This is problematic as a seizure can cause re-bleeding or expansion of the bleed.

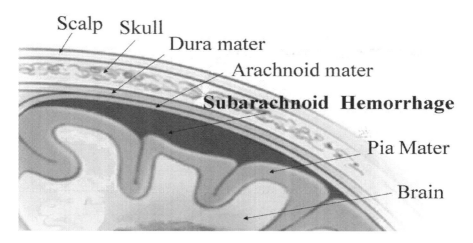

Patients are often brought to an emergency room under the influence of drugs or alcohol, especially late at night and in the early morning hours. Furthermore, young adults typically do not have head bleeds or strokes. What exactly the healthcare team working that night had been told will never be known, but they thought the patient's drinking and drug use led to his confusion. Had they done a CT, they likely would have seen the blood on the scan and initiated transfer. One might argue the CT scan should have been done on his arrival; however, it's impractical to scan every patient who walks into an ED, especially when there appears to be an obvious cause of the patient's symptoms. The costs involved and the radiation exposure risk to the patient must be considered.

The Flight Out and Game Plan:

It was mid-morning, and our flight team had flown to a public relations event. We were all enjoying a pancake breakfast when our pagers began beeping. The pilots accepted the flight and we walked to the helicopter and lifted 5 minutes later. The hospital was about 80 miles away, or a 25 minute helicopter flight from our location with a helipad on site. In the air, we radioed for a patient update and were notified that our patient was a 32 year old male. The diagnosis of subarachnoid hemorrhage had been confirmed, and he was reported to be drowsy but still alert. The patient's heart rate was a bit below normal in the 50s, he had a high blood pressure of 182/95, and normal oxygen levels.

Because young athletes sometimes have a slower than normal heart rate, we thought his slow rate might have been normal. This was still concerning, though, because high intracranial pressures, created from the bleeding, can also cause a decreased heart rate from increased pressure on the vagus nerve. The vagus nerve plays an important role at regulating heart rate. Young men his age typically do not have systolic blood pressures (top number) in the 180s and this indicated a potential high intracranial pressure, likely contributing to his altered mental status. As intracranial pressure increases, patients become progressively more confused due to altered blood flow to brain cells. The body attempts to compensate for this with a higher blood pressure to perfuse the brain. Unfortunately, this can make the bleeding worse.

We had several priorities for transporting this patient. We needed to find out if our patient had any potential bleeding problems so we could relay this information to the accepting hospital. Other priorities included decreasing any elevations of intracranial pressure to improve brain cell function, lowering his blood pressure to reduce the size of the bleed, and ensuring he could protect his airway and breathe. All of this had to be done rapidly because it was essential to get him to a higher level of care as fast as possible. If we had time, we might also give a drug to prevent the potential seizures sometimes seen with this type of head bleed.

The game plan was to give mannitol if he showed significant signs of confusion and to lower his systolic blood pressure to around 140 with a drug called hydralazine. Although IV medications other than hydralazine are sometimes given to lower blood pressure for this condition, they might slow his heart rate further and his rate was already below normal. Mannitol is a drug often given in severe head bleeds to remove fluid from the brain into the vascular system. As the fluid leaves the brain, intracranial pressure should decrease. We planned to assess his airway status and, if he could not breathe adequately on his own, place a breathing tube. To prepare for the worst and be ready for intubation, we calculated the doses of any drug we might give. Twenty minutes later we landed, and a security guard escorted us to the emergency department.

The Transport:

As we entered the emergency department, the physician on duty met us at the door and walked with us to our patient's room. The physician briefly informed us about the situation then went to see another patient. In the hospital bed lay a younger-looking man in a deep sleep. He seemed quite a bit drowsier than we had expected, still hypertensive with a blood pressure of 178/101 and a heart rate in the low

50s. My partner gave hydralazine to lower his blood pressure and I began to assess our patient.

I called him by his first name and he slowly opened his eyes halfway, but only for a second, then fell back to sleep. I yelled his name again and got the same response. "Sir," I said in a loud voice..."Sir." "Sir...what's your name?" He slowly opened his eyes, looked at me, said something incomprehensible, and fell back asleep. I put my hands in his and yelled for him to squeeze my hands. He squeezed my hands. I asked him to wiggle his toes; he wiggled his toes. Although barely arousable, he could at least still follow simple commands.

The patient only had one IV, which was not enough to safely attempt the transport. His symptoms suggested that his intracranial pressures were too high and he likely would soon need a breathing tube. As I placed two more IVs, my partner started a mannitol IV infusion and placed it in a pressure bag. The pressure bag acts to squeeze the drug into the body, decreasing its infusion time. We hoped the mannitol might relieve the pressure on his brain by pulling fluid from the intracranial space, and as a result, our patient might waken enough to avoid intubation. This was not certain, though, and he might continue to deteriorate during the transport, so I asked the nurse if she would call for the physician. I did not want the patient to crash in mid-flight and I valued the physician's opinion.

My gut feeling was to place the breathing tube before transport, but sometimes physicians feel as though we "step on their toes," and take offense if we do things like that without their consent. The doc and I talked for a few minutes and he said the patient had been like that all night. I sensed he just wanted us out of there and thought to myself, *if he has been like this all night, it only confirms the need for a tube.* But I refrained from saying anything to avoid offending him. I reassessed the situation and while our patient appeared extremely sleepy, he still maintained his airway, although only marginally. If he needed tubed in flight, we would just have to do it then. In the meantime, my partner started a drug to prevent possible seizures which sometimes occur after intracranial bleeding. We put him on our transport cot and left the bedside.

Loading our patient into the aircraft proved to be the only normal part of the transport. We loaded and secured him inside the aircraft as the pilots began their startup checklists. While lifting off from the helipad, we checked another blood pressure to see if the medication we had given worked. The BP cuff cycled and read 172/94, still too high, and we gave another dose of hydralazine. Once at a cruising altitude, we rechecked the pressure…148/82: it had finally lowered near our target of 140 systolic.

The mannitol we had given to remove fluid from the brain had finished infusing. The fluid from his brain and other cells in his body had now filled his bladder and I would soon regret not placing a foley catheter before we left. Had I placed a foley, urine would be in a bag and not his bladder. Out of nowhere, having no idea where he was, he opened his eyes, sat up, and yelled "I have to take a piss!"

He aggressively tried to unbuckle himself from the cot, struggling to get out. But in a helicopter, 2,500 feet above the ground, there was nowhere for him to go and this behavior put the entire crew in danger. We rushed to find a urinal but it was too late. Our patient pulled his pants partly down and began to urinate all over himself with some of it going about the cabin. Not able to find a urinal, we placed a small garbage bag in a position which would catch most of the urine. After all of this, as quickly as it started, he laid his head back on the cot and closed his eyes. We left the bag between his legs in case this scenario repeated itself, but this proved to be only one more glitch in the transport. Things would get much worse.

Patients with high intracranial pressures sometimes vomit, so we gave a medication intended to relieve nausea and vomiting, hoping to prevent this. We had already been urinated on and preferred to avoid displaying vomit on our flight suits. Less than 10 minutes after giving the medication, he again began to sit up, attempting to get off the cot. I noticed retching movements from his chest and knew he was about to puke, so I reached to further raise the head of the bed, hoping he would not aspirate into his lungs.

My partner grabbed an emesis bag but we could not convey to our patient to put it over his mouth, nor did he comprehend what to do. He sat straight up in the aircraft and threw-up. He then began kicking and reaching for both my partner and I, trying to undo the buckles that secured him to the cot. We tried to suction the vomit from his mouth but he just pushed our hand away. By this time we were on final approach for landing. This was unsafe and my partner and I agreed to sedate, paralyze, and intubate him once on the ground. We began to get everything ready.

We landed, and all of a sudden he became calm again. His vitals were stable. He was breathing and maintaining his airway. Since we were so close to the unit he had been assigned to by this point, we decided it might be safer to delay placing the breathing tube for 2 or 3 minutes. There is no back up on the helipad if something goes wrong and we thought we could safely make it to the accepting unit. Once there, they could complete a neurological exam and decide if he needed to emergently go to the operating room and then intubate if needed.

After unloading our transport cot from the helicopter, we met a security guard designated to escort us to the intensive care unit our patient was going. But, since we had been to this hospital many times before, and our patient remained calm, we told the guard he did not need to go with us and proceeded into the hospital. This proved to be a big mistake. The mannitol must have worked because he indeed woke up as we travelled down the hospital hallway. Upon entering the intensive care unit, pandemonium erupted.

In the middle of the unit, he sat up once again and turned his body, trying to get off the cot. My partner and I tried to hold him down as other staff came to help us. We struggled to keep him from falling off the cot and quickly moved next to his designated bed. By this time, it seemed like the entire unit had gathered in the room, so with the help of several nurses and the accepting physician, we moved him to the bed. He was yelling, confused, and doing all in his power to get out of the bed. At this point, it became obvious that to protect the safety of all the medical staff and the patient, we had to sedate and paralyze him. Doing this, however, meant we also needed to completely take over his breathing. Feeling partially responsible for having not insisted on doing this at the sending hospital, I moved to the head of the bed to place the breathing tube. I looked at the doc and asked if I could place the tube, since I was already in the ideal position, and he said okay.

We had brought all our equipment, had already calculated our drug doses, and had everything ready to go, since we had planned to do this earlier. The hospital nurses fought to hold the man down while my partner gave the medications. It only took seconds for the drugs to take effect and he went into a deep sleep and became completely lifeless. I placed a mask over his nose and mouth then manually breathed for him for several minutes with an ambu bag. Next, I opened his mouth, gently inserted a laryngoscope, and manipulated it to visualize his vocal cords.

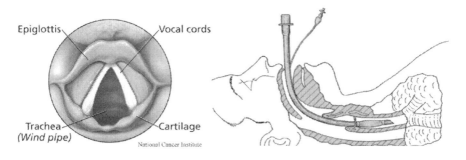

I could barely see my target, but managed to place the tube between his cords, and into the trachea, without too much difficulty. After confirming the tube was in the right position, we connected him to the hospital ventilator. The nurses then started an IV infusion which would continue to keep him in an induced coma.

Finally the trip was over with. I thanked the nurses and accepting physician for all their help and we flew back to base, restocked our medications and equipment, and cleaned the aircraft. Now all I wanted to do was take a shower, but we had 7 more hours left in our shift. I went to the restroom at our base and had just finished washing my hands, arms, and face when I my pager went off again.

The Outcome:

Our patient needed to emergently go to the operating room, where an aneurysm was found and coiled. Coiling is a minimally invasive endovascular procedure to treat aneurysms. During coiling, very small coils are filled into an aneurysm, stopping blood from flowing into it, yet allowing blood to flow freely through the normal arteries. He had a full neurological recovery and was later discharged home.

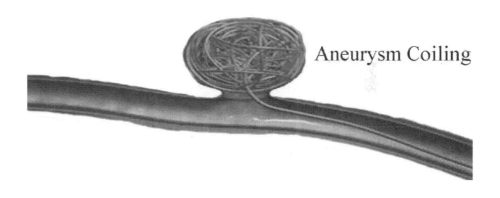

Aneurysm Coiling

Take Home Points:

For the Nurse or EMS Provider:

A subarachnoid hemorrhage (SAH) bleeds between the pial and arachnoid membranes of the brain and is most often caused by a ruptured aneurysm- about 80-85% of the time.

SAH is typically diagnosed with head CT showing blood in the subarachnoid space. However, SAH blood is not always seen on CT and if CT is normal, a lumbar puncture is usually done to look for red blood cells in the cerebral spinal fluid.

A major complication of SAH is re-bleeding. The immediate goal is to prevent elevations in blood pressure and intracranial pressure until the aneurysm is secured with a coil or clip. This is why any diagnosed SAH must be transported to a neurosurgical center capable of these interventions.

Recommendations for target systolic blood pressure vary and there is no clear evidence identifying an ideal number. Hypotension can increase the risk of infarction but if patient is alert, SBP < 140 mm Hg is typical[2]. It is important to prevent hypotension and carefully monitor these patients for signs of cerebral hypoperfusion, which may result if blood pressure is too low.

We gave mannitol early in the transport because we thought his intracranial pressures were high, causing his altered mental status. Mannitol pulled excess fluid from the cranium, along with other areas of the body, and he began to waken. This fluid went to the bladder, which contributed to our mid-air urinal episode. Although there was quite a bit to do on this transport, in retrospect, I would have asked the nurse to place a foley catheter while we were placing IV lines and hanging meds.

Mannitol will pull fluid from the body into the vascular space and can cause acute pulmonary edema…especially in heart failure patients.

Elevating the head of the bed and keeping the head from turning to improve venous drainage will help lower ICP.

Increased pressure in the brain/skull is often associated with projectile vomiting.

For the Public:

Do not use drugs or drink excessively. Not only do they alter your thinking, increasing your chance of accidental injury, they can cause long-term health problems and cloud the picture for health care professionals when a real emergency exists.

Subarachnoid hemorrhage symptoms can include a sudden headache, usually severe, often described as the "worst headache of one's life, thunderclap headache, or a severe blow to the head". Other symptoms can be a stiff neck, nausea, vomiting, slurred speech, confusion or impaired consciousness, occasionally seizures, difficulty lifting an eyelid, sharp increase in blood pressure, vision changes, difficulty speaking, sudden confusion, problems walking, or a severe sudden headache different from other headaches.

WHAT HAPPENED IN VEGAS?

Setting:

Most people who visit Las Vegas have memories of casinos, neon lights, slot machines, grand food buffets, and amazing entertainment. My recollections of Vegas are quite different. I recall a patient transport: being pressed for time and a patient with severe heart failure, low blood pressure, and kidney failure. This is a story of a 65-year old male we transported from Las Vegas to the other side of the country in severe heart failure and in dire need of a heart transplant.

This man had a history of multiple and major heart complications, which originated from coronary artery disease (CAD). In his mid-40s, he suffered his first heart attack and underwent three-vessel coronary artery bypass grafting (CABG). Then in his late-50s, two of the bypass grafts became occluded and he had a second major heart attack that required two stents within the grafts. His heart attacks caused severe structural heart changes and its function had deteriorated to one third of the normal heart. His ejection fraction, the percentage of blood emptied from his left ventricle with each heartbeat, was only 20%.

After the second heart attack, he lived independently at home for several years until he experienced recurring shortness of breath. To optimize what little heart function he had left, a biventricular pacer had been placed. He was doing better until six months later when he presented to a small medical center in Las Vegas with persistent weakness and shortness of breath, even at rest.

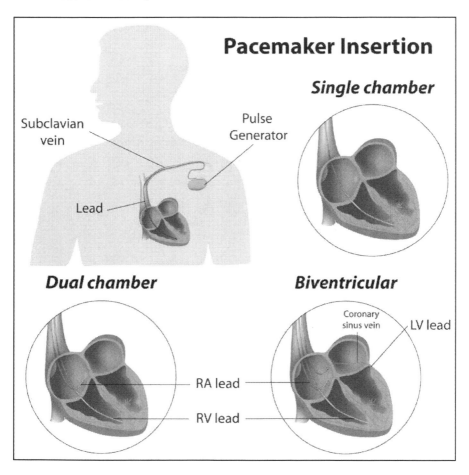

Pacemaker Insertion

Single chamber

Subclavian vein

Pulse Generator

Lead

Dual chamber

Biventricular

Coronary sinus vein

LV lead

RA lead

RV lead

He was admitted to the hospital and treated for acute congestive heart failure. The hospital gave the diuretic Lasix, hoping this might remove excessive fluid thought to have accumulated in his lungs. Blood testing indicated that he had suffered from yet another heart attack. An echocardiogram showed his heart function had declined yet again and his ejection fraction was now only 5-10%. This meant that, of all the blood sitting in the left ventricle before his heart contracted, only 5-10% of it left the heart with each contraction. His kidneys began to weaken due to lack of blood flow from his poor heart function.

The hospital in Las Vegas made several medication adjustments attempting to improve his cardiac output, but his kidneys continued to fail and he would soon need dialysis. Six days after being admitted to the hospital, the physicians managing his care in Las Vegas thought that transporting him to an institution capable of heart transplant was his only chance of survival. Unfortunately, the medical center that accepted him for evaluation was on the other side of the country. Our flight team was requested to transport him there by fixed wing aircraft.

Everyday Language Of What Might Be Going On:

Heart failure is a term which basically means the cardiac output is not meeting the needs of the body. There are two different types of heart failure, left-sided and right-sided. Left-sided heart failure is far more common than right and often contributes to the development of right-sided heart failure. Each can cause unique symptoms. A person in heart failure can, and often does, have a degree of both left- and right-sided failure with symptoms of both. To understand why these symptoms occur requires a general idea of how and why blood flows through the body.

Every organ in the body consists of microscopic cells which need oxygen to live. The byproduct of cellular metabolism is carbon dioxide. The body must get oxygen to the cells and remove carbon dioxide created by the cells to survive. If it cannot do this, the cells of the organ will deteriorate and die. The body uses the heart, lungs, and blood to accomplish this and the process occurs in the following manner.

1. When you inhale, oxygen from the atmosphere moves into the lungs.

2. Once in the lungs, oxygen travels to the blood and then to the left side of the heart. This happens at the same time carbon dioxide leaves the blood and travels into the lungs.

3. Oxygenated blood leaves the left ventricle with each heartbeat and travels through the aorta, into the arteries, and eventually reaches the tissues of the body.

4. Once at the tissue cells, oxygen moves to the cells, while carbon dioxide moves from the cells to the blood.

5. After this exchange of oxygen and carbon dioxide, the blood then enters the venous system.

6. The carbon dioxide-filled blood is now heading to the right side of the heart via the venous system as the heart beats.

7. The blood that travels to the right side of the heart contains less oxygen and more carbon dioxide. It is pumped to the lungs by the right ventricle.

8. As blood passes by the lungs, the excess carbon dioxide moves from the blood to the lungs, leaves the body when you exhale, and the cycle repeats.

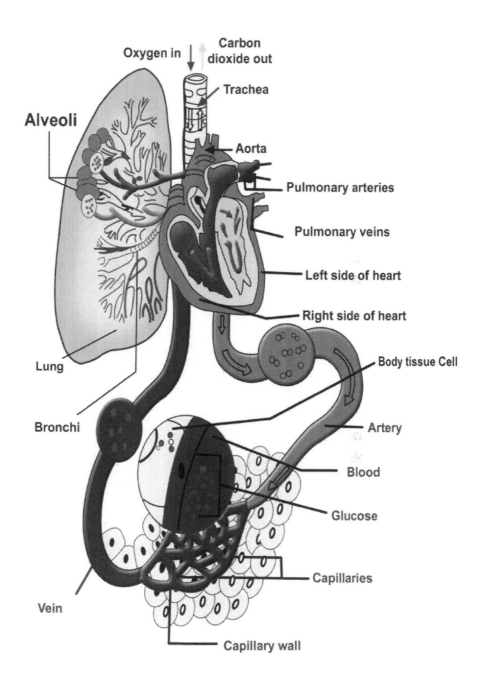

Oxygen in

Carbon dioxide out

Trachea

Alveoli

Aorta

Pulmonary arteries

Pulmonary veins

Left side of heart

Right side of heart

Body tissue Cell

Lung

Artery

Bronchi

Blood

Glucose

Capillaries

Vein

Capillary wall

Without the lungs, heart, or blood, cells cannot get oxygen nor remove carbon dioxide. In right sided heart failure, the right side of the heart is not effectively pumping blood to the lungs. Blood can then "back up" and cause congestion in the liver, gastrointestinal tract, and limbs. An example of this "fluid back up" is the edema sometimes seen in the ankles or other parts of the body. Also, the right ventricle may be unable to pump blood efficiently to the lungs and to the left ventricle leading to shortness of breath and/or hypotension.

The left ventricle is the "powerhouse" of the heart. This is the part of the heart most responsible for blood flow to the body. The left ventricle does not pump adequately for those with left-sided heart failure. As the volume of blood the heart pumps with each heartbeat (ejection fraction) declines, instead of moving blood to the body, blood can back up in the lungs. This creates a higher than normal intravascular pulmonary pressure, forcing fluid to leak from the blood into the lungs. The fluid in the lungs obstructs gas exchange and patients may become short of breath or cough up frothy sputum.

In severe left-sided heart failure, the left ventricle is not strong enough to move blood to the tissues. These tissues, therefore, cannot get enough oxygen or remove carbon dioxide. If blood flow to these tissues is poor enough, they can die. To compensate for this, the kidneys sense the decrease in blood flow and attempt to retain fluid. In dehydration, keeping fluid is helpful. But in heart failure, the added fluid causes further congestion and worsens the problem.

There are several goals of treatment and medications prescribed for patients in heart failure. ACE inhibitors or other anti-hypertensive medications are used to reduce blood pressure. This creates less resistance in the arteries and makes it easier for the heart to pump effectively. It's also important to prevent too much stimulation of the heart; thus, beta blockers are often prescribed. Finally, diuretics are ordered to help remove the excess fluid retained by the kidneys. When heart failure is severe enough, other medications or mechanical devices are sometimes used to improve blood flow to the body.

This patient had reached a point at which his heart only pumped a minimal volume of blood, leading to extreme shortness of breath and kidney failure. Medications no longer were enough for this man. A biventricular pacer had been placed as a last ditch effort to improve his cardiac function by triggering a heart contraction at an optimal time. Unfortunately, this only helped for a short period. His heart had become too weak and his only chance of long-term survival was a heart transplant.

The Flight Out and Game Plan:

At 7 o'clock in the morning, my 24 hour on-call shift had just started and I woke up to an obnoxiously loud beeping from my pager. I reached over to my nightstand, grabbed the pager and read, "patient transfer from Las Vegas to east coast, lift time 0830." I climbed out of bed, took a five minute shower, put on my flight suit, and grabbed a cup of coffee before heading out the door. While driving to the airport, I called our dispatch center to inform them I was on my way. I asked for a patient status update, wanting to know about the patient and what to expect for the transport. Unfortunately, the information given to me was no longer current.

A separate crew had tried to complete the transport the prior night, but their plane had broken down after stopping for fuel and they never made it to the patient. I received the same report given to the previous crew. At that time, the patient was stable and he had an oxygen requirement of 2 liters nasal cannula. This is a minimal amount of oxygen and often indicates an uneventful transport. He had a normal heart rate and his blood pressure 14 hours ago was 96/58. This is a bit low, but a lower than normal blood pressure is expected with a patient in heart failure, especially if they are on anti-hypertensive medications. I asked why he was being transferred so far. When they told me the transfer was for a possible heart transplant, things didn't make sense. If he needed a transplant, why did he have to fly so far, and why was he so stable? I'd later find out he was not so stable and this transport would not be routine.

I made it to the airport by 8 o'clock. My partner and I used back-up equipment since the prior crew had taken the primary set. We verified we had all the essential gear and that none of our medications had expired, and we loaded everything onto the jet plane. The pilots gave us our normal flight briefing and informed us the flight was too far to fly direct. We needed to stop for fuel on the way out, but might be able to fly back nonstop from Las Vegas depending on conditions. A direct flight with our patient on board meant less time for something to go wrong, so this was potentially good news. Since we had to stop for fuel, I planned on calling the sending hospital in Las Vegas for a patient update and to give them an estimated time of arrival. We lifted right on schedule at 8:30 AM and I took a short nap on the flight out.

Two hours later, we landed for fuel and encountered the first glitch of the transport. Our pilots informed us we would have less than two hours to be back in the air once we landed in Las Vegas. If it took longer, we would be forced to stay the night in Vegas and finish the transport the next day. This might be a huge problem, since the hospital was a 30 minute drive from the airport. If we had an extended bedside time, we would be forced to leave our patient at the hospital for another day.

I walked into the airport terminal and noticed our other crew, who had broken down the prior night. They looked exhausted, having been up the entire previous night. We spoke briefly and they told me what they knew about the patient. I wished them a safe flight home and went to a private location to call the sending hospital, which is when I first realized this transport might be challenging.

I called the hospital in Vegas and spoke with the nurse taking care of our patient that day. Based on the report she gave me, he was not doing well. The nurse had trouble getting a blood pressure, with the last one reading 72/48. Systolic blood pressures (top number) below 90 are concerning because organs of the body usually require at least 90 to function. The patient's creatinine was continuing to rise, and he had stopped urinating. Creatinine is removed by the kidneys, and is a measurement of kidney function. When creatinine rises, it suggests the kidneys are not working properly. Another more immediate way to gauge kidney function is to monitor urine output and, since he no longer made urine, it appeared as if his kidneys were failing.

After the nurse told me the patient's blood pressure, I wondered why the hospital allowed it to stay so low and if his mental status was normal. If he was confused, this might indicate his brain was not getting enough blood. I asked the nurse how his mental status was and she told me he was alert and normally oriented. Although apparently still perfusing his brain, it looked as if his heart was not pumping enough blood to his kidneys. I then asked about several other electrolytes regulated by the kidneys, specifically his potassium level. If potassium is too high or low, serious cardiac arrhythmias, or even complete cardiac standstill, can result. The last thing I wanted on the 4.5 hour flight to the accepting hospital was to deal with cardiac arrhythmias. Unfortunately, since the hospital had expected the flight team the night before, none of these labs had been sent and none were current.

Surprisingly, the patient only had one small intravenous (IV) line in his arm, and no IV infusions running that might help increase his cardiac function and/or blood pressure. Kidneys cannot survive without a decent blood pressure to perfuse them and this patient needed as much kidney function as possible before the heart transplant. Many of the anti-rejection medications given after transplant can cause kidney damage, so having optimal renal function is essential. Without it, he might not even be considered for transplant. Hearts are not a common commodity and surgeons are reluctant to transplant those unlikely to have a good outcome. This hospital should have been doing everything possible to maximize cardiac output. Instead, they could not get an accurate blood pressure, no IV infusions that might help improve his cardiac function were running, and he didn't have a central line to infuse them.

Medical institutions are not equal in terms of quality of patient care. To better monitor and correct this man's cardiac dysfunction, it sounded like he needed to be in an intensive care unit. There, they could place an arterial line for continuous blood pressure monitoring and a central line to infuse medications that might help increase his cardiac output and blood pressure. To this hospital's credit, they realized the patient needed a higher level of care and they initiated transfer.

I thanked the nurse for her time and told her we planned to arrive at the hospital in about 3 hours. Before hanging up the phone, I explained our time dilemma and requested that the hospital place a special type of IV called a peripherally inserted central catheter, commonly called a PICC line. I also asked if they might check the electrolytes while we were en route. I didn't feel comfortable flying him with only one IV and no central access to infuse medications. Although we are capable of placing these, we didn't have enough time, and if we waited until the next day to transfer him, his kidney function would only worsen.

The fuel stop was quick and we were airborne 20 minutes later. I updated my partner about the report the nurse had given me and we discussed what our plan would be once in Las Vegas. We could either take a layover day and finish the trip the next day, or be rushed and get our patient to a higher level of care sooner. Slot machines and food buffets sounded fun at the time, but the patient needed transferred that day. His condition would only worsen with time so we decided to do everything possible to avoid an additional delay for the transport. During the next leg of the flight, we enjoyed an amazing view as we flew over the Great Salt Lake, the Grand Canyon, and the Hoover Dam. Two-and-a-half hours later we landed in Las Vegas and it was time for us to shift into high gear.

An ambulance was waiting on us and pulled next to our plane and the pilots reminded us of our time limit. We now had 1 hour and 40 minutes to be back. I took one of their cell phone numbers and gave them mine just in case any issues should occur, told them we'd be back on time or I'd call if we couldn't make it. We loaded our equipment into the squad, explained the time dilemma to the ambulance driver, and asked him to "run hot." "Hot" is emergency slang for as fast as possible with lights and sirens. The driver nodded his head, said yes, and we sped to the accepting hospital with lights and sirens blaring.

As we raced to the hospital, I again called the nurse taking care of the patient for an updated report over the phone to save time at bedside. Our patient was still alert but a bit sleepier. I became somewhat concerned about blood perfusion to his brain. The nurse continued to have trouble obtaining blood pressures, with the last pressure of 78/42. Thankfully, the hospital had placed the PICC line I requested and resent the chemistry labs. Aside from his creatinine, which was still rising, his electrolytes were only slightly abnormal and we did not expect any problems in that regard. But if our patient's heart could not pump enough blood to his body, the transport might be problematic.

The PICC line allowed us to safely begin IV infusions which might improve his cardiac function and improve blood flow to his organs, especially his kidneys. We planned to put the patient on our monitor, quickly place an arterial line, move him to the cot, and then leave. An arterial line is a tiny catheter similar to an IV that sits inside the artery. This allows clinicians to more accurately monitor blood pressures with each heartbeat. If possible, we wanted to know his exact and continuous blood pressure, especially if giving medications to improve them.

We pulled into the small hospital almost 25 minutes later. The ambulance driver told us the drive back to the airport might be a few minutes longer because of traffic. We estimated the ride back would take 35 minutes and it would take another 10 minutes to load him in the jet. This allowed us to spend no more than 25 minutes at the hospital. We unloaded the cot from the ambulance with our equipment secured to it and asked the driver to remind us 5 minutes before we needed to go. We quickly walked to our patient's unit, located on the other side of the hospital, and by the time we arrived there we had only 20 minutes to get everything done.

The Transport:

I walked into the room and met our patient for the first time. He appeared somewhat sleepy, but in talking with him it reassured me to see he was alert and attentive. This signified his blood pressure was high enough to at least provide blood flow to his brain. Unfortunately, this was not the case for his extremities. His arms and legs were cool and his pulses could barely be felt. When I asked him how he felt, he just said extremely weak. I asked him if he had any trouble breathing or chest pain and he responded no.

My partner placed him on our monitor and cycled the blood pressure cuff, but it could not take a reading because his pressure was so low. I explained to our patient that we needed to start medications which might help increase blood flow to his extremities and, more importantly, his kidneys. I told him to do this safely it was necessary to have an arterial line and explained briefly what it was. He agreed to the procedure and I began to set up the supplies needed to place it. In the meantime, my partner took a manual blood pressure the old fashion way, using a sphygmomanometer and stethoscope. Unfortunately, this method of obtaining a blood pressure can be inaccurate. His systolic pressure, we thought, was somewhere between 70 and 80.

By the time I had assessed him and gotten everything ready for the arterial line, we had only ten minutes until our departure time. I cleaned and prepped his wrist and inserted an access needle towards his radial artery. His pulses were so weak, I was not sure if I felt his pulse or mine, so I aimed in the proper anatomical direction. Sometimes these catheters go right in, but other times it takes a lot of manipulation to find the artery. If ever I needed a procedure to go smoothly, this was the time. I tried for several minutes, gently moving the needle forward and backward at various angles, but could not find the artery. The ambulance driver called out our 5-minute warning and I had to wrap up, even without the arterial line.

Now came a crucial decision point of the transport. Do we leave the hospital without being able to obtain an accurate blood pressure, or plan to come back the next day with ample time to place an arterial line? If we left without the line, we could only hope our cuff pressures would read and we might have to guess at what his true blood pressure really was. If we waited to transport him, his kidney function would worsen and reduce the likelihood of a good outcome. My partner and I briefly talked this over and decided our patient couldn't wait. He needed transported today. I'd just have to try the line again in the air or ambulance.

I put the needles I had used in the sharps container and threw the other materials in the trash. We lifted our patient onto the transport cot and fastened the buckles. The nurse brought the patient's medical records into the room and we were ready to go. Before we left, I asked the nurse if I could have an arterial line kit since I had used the only one we carry in our transport bag. There is another kit on the plane, but since it had been so long since we originally checked our equipment in the morning, I was unsure if I remembered seeing it. The nurse kindly gave me a kit and we departed the bedside. At this point, we had 50 minutes to get back to the airport and load the patient on the plane.

As fast as we had walked into the hospital, we hurried back to the ambulance and loaded our patient into the squad. My partner and I jumped in the back, secured our patient, and began the return trip to the airport with lights and sirens running. The patient's heart rate was in the low 100s, a few beats higher than normal, but still an acceptable rate. He seemed to be oxygenating appropriately but we could not get a blood pressure.

We knew his heart at least still perfused his brain since he conversed with us, but how much blood was reaching his kidneys and other organs? With five or six hours to monitor him, we still needed an arterial line to determine his exact hemodynamic status. We debated trying this again in the ambulance, but our next attempt might be our last. It was too bumpy in the squad, so we agreed to save our kit and try in the air, heading back toward the east coast. In the meantime, we started an IV drug infusion called norepinephrine, assuming his blood pressure was low. This drug can help the heart generate a stronger contraction and raise the blood pressure.

Soon after starting norepinephrine, we finally got a cuff blood pressure reading... 91/54. This was somewhat of a relief. Although not great, a systolic blood pressure in the 90s is better than 60s, 70s, or 80s. I called our pilots and gave them a 15-minute estimated time of arrival (ETA) so they would have everything ready for us to load the patient. I also contacted the cardiologist at the admitting hospital across the country to ask which drugs he preferred we start if our patient needed more medications to support his blood pressure. We had several drugs to choose from in our transport supply, but I wanted clarification about his drugs of choice. If we needed to start them in flight, I preferred to use his favored medications.

The cardiologist and I discussed our patient's fluid status and whether to give him more IV fluid or attempt to remove some with a diuretic. Giving a fluid bolus to a weak heart might force fluid into the lungs and create unwanted respiratory problems, including the possible need for a breathing tube. Conversely, if he had too much fluid already, his heart might be overstretched, and removing fluid might improve his blood pressure. But his pressure was already low and a diuretic might make it worse if this was not the problem. We had no room for error and concluded it best to avoid giving either IV fluid or a diuretic. The safest choice seemed to be to attempt improvement of his cardiac function and blood pressure with vasoactive medications.

Although we could try and maximize his cardiac function, there was no guarantee any of this would work. His heart was, after all, only one-tenth the strength of a normal heart. We rechecked his blood pressure just before arriving at the airport and his systolic pressure had dipped to 80s. Unsure if this was even accurate, we delayed increasing the norepinephrine until after trying to place an arterial line since he was alert and still talking to us.

We arrived at the airport with 20 minutes to spare. Our pilots had set the aircraft cot on the tarmac, waiting for us to load our patient. The squad pulled next to the jet and we loaded our unused equipment into the aircraft cabin. We pulled the stretcher off the squad and rolled it next to the aircraft cot. With the pilots' help, we lifted the patient and fastened him securely to the cot, with the monitor and pump resting between his legs. One pilot and I jumped into the plane, while my partner and the other pilot set up the ramp used to load patients in the cabin. Together, the pilot outside, my partner, and the crew who drove us to the hospital lifted our patient onto the ramp and we maneuvered him into the plane.

The pilots closed and locked the aircraft door, moved to the front of the plane, and prepared for takeoff. While they did this, my partner and I finished securing our patient and equipment, then positioned our monitor and IV pumps so we could easily see them. I sat in a seat which gave me the best position to place the arterial line once we reached a stable altitude and fastened my seat belt. Taxiing down the runway, we took another blood pressure, but again there was no reading. The pilots were cleared for takeoff. They looked back to us and asked if we were ready, and we gave them a nod in the affirmative. The engines revved louder and louder, the pilots released the breaks, and we went speeding down the runway.

We took off and began ascending to cruising altitude. Objects on the earth became smaller and smaller as we swayed in the air. Within a couple minutes, it became smooth enough for another try at the arterial line. I positioned our patient's right arm on top of a transport bag and taped his hand so it would not move. I unbuckled my seatbelt, numbed the underside of his wrist with a drug called lidocaine, opened the arterial line kit, and put on sterile gloves. Next, I cleaned and sterilized his wrist and grabbed a catheter used to access the artery. This is similar to an IV, with a small needle inside a plastic catheter. His pulse was faint. Above the area I thought was his pulse, I inserted the catheter into his wrist, towards the artery, and saw a flash of bright red blood come out the back.

A sense of relief came over me, since this looked to be arterial blood. I removed the needle, leaving only the catheter in the artery. As the needle came out, pulsating blood flowed from the catheter hub. I gently inserted part of a sterile wire through the catheter and into his artery and removed the small catheter. Now half of the wire was in the artery and I held the other half in my hand. I grabbed a larger and sturdier catheter, placed the wire through its lumen, advanced it into the artery, and pulled the wire out. Pulsating blood came out of the larger catheter as I connected it to our hemodynamic monitoring line. Success...we now viewed an exact blood pressure with each heartbeat.

His arterial pressures were only 60 to 70 systolic, so we increased the norepinephrine IV infusion to its maximum recommended dose. This brought his systolic blood pressure to the low 80s, which was still not adequate. Now with an arterial line in place to precisely measure his blood pressure, we started a dobutamine IV infusion, which the accepting cardiologist had suggested during our conversation. This drug is used to maximize cardiac output, giving the heart a stronger contraction. On occasion, though, it can sometimes lower blood pressure by slightly dilating the arterial system. I had been advised by the cardiologist, however, that even if this happened we should leave it running and add another IV infusion called dopamine. I hoped further medications would not be required, though. After starting the dobutamine, and with the norepinephrine infusing at the maximum recommended dose, we finally had a systolic blood pressure just above 90.

We reached a cruising altitude of 35,000 feet and our patient said he had trouble breathing. This sometimes happens at higher altitudes because the air is thinner with less available oxygen. To avoid this, aircraft can pressurize the cabin to lower altitudes, but this slows the speed of the aircraft and causes a higher rate of fuel consumption. My partner grabbed an oxygen mask and put it on our patient while I called our pilots on the aircraft phone and asked them to pressurize the cabin. This improved his breathing but meant we now had a longer flight time and needed to stop for fuel.

Over the next two hours, his systolic blood pressures fluctuated between 85 and 90. While monitoring our patient, we went through his medical records more thoroughly even though his most concerning illness was obvious: poor cardiac function. When his pressure consistently stayed in the low 80s we increased the dose of the dobutamine, but we eventually reached its maximum dose. With 3 hours left in the transport, we were on maximal doses of the first two drugs recommended by the cardiologist. Although we wanted his systolic pressure above 90, his extremely weak heart just could not achieve that, and 85 to 90 might be the best his heart would pump. Every few minutes, we asked our patient a question or made conversation, just to verify he still perfused his brain. Except for his low blood pressure, he remained stable. We landed in the Midwest to refuel.

Once on the ground, I called the cardiologist I had spoken with earlier to update him on our patient's status and give an estimated time of arrival. I told the doc we had placed the arterial line but our patient's pressures remained low, even on norepinephrine and dobutamine at their max doses. I relayed that we had been accepting systolic blood pressures of 85 to 90. I also verified his drugs of choice in case we needed a third agent to increase his blood pressure and asked at what pressure he wanted it started. We discussed this for several minutes and agreed that if our patient's systolic blood pressure remained under 80 consistently, we would add a drug called dopamine. I hoped to not have to resort to dopamine, however, since this drug occasionally triggers cardiac arrhythmias.

After 15 minutes on the ground, we departed for our destination city with approximately a 2 hour flight time. 30 minutes into the second leg of our patient's journey, his systolic blood pressures dropped consistently into the high 70s. Since he was still at the maximum dose of both norepinephrine and dobutamine, we were forced to add a third medication, dopamine. This raised his systolic blood pressure to the low 90s and they remained between 85 and 90 for the rest of the flight. Now I needed to prepare our patient for what might happen once at the accepting hospital.

While on the phone with the accepting cardiologist at the airport, he had told me they planned to place an intra-aortic balloon pump (IABP) as soon as we arrived at the hospital. I explained to our patient what this was and how it might help him. An IABP is a mechanical device in which a catheter with a balloon is placed in the aorta to improve coronary blood flow and cardiac output. When the heart is relaxed, the balloon inflates to help increase coronary blood flow. Just before each heart contraction, the balloon deflates as blood is ejected from the left ventricle, reducing the workload of the heart.

For the rest of the transport, we tried minor adjustments in drug dosing, but his systolic blood pressures did not get much higher than 85. Even though his pressure was better than when we began the transport, there was no guarantee his kidneys were perfusing. We landed at our destination city, and unloading our patient proved to be more challenging than loading him. With our 3 pumps, cardiac monitor, and oxygen tank situated around his body, we inched the aircraft stretcher off the plane and set it on the tarmac. Next, we positioned the awaiting ambulance cot next to the stretcher and moved each piece of equipment. Finally, with the help of two paramedics assigned to drive us to the hospital, we lifted the patient to the ambulance cot and loaded him into the squad.

Faced with only a short 15 to 20 minute drive to the accepting hospital, the most difficult parts of the transport were now behind us. Provided there were no unforeseen events, it looked as if the transport would be a success. There were no major complications aside from the continually low blood pressure. While we drove to the awaiting hospital, I called the cardiologist to give our estimated time of arrival and informed him of the third IV infusion we had started. He said a team would be ready in a procedure room to place the intra-aortic balloon pump and advised us to take our patient directly there. Twenty minutes later, we arrived at the hospital and took him to the designated room. The team was waiting on us and we updated them about the flight and gave a brief report. Then we helped lift our patient to the procedure table as the nurses transferred each IV infusion to their pumps and connected their monitoring equipment.

We left his medical records with the secretary before saying good bye to our patient and telling him he was in good hands. He thanked us for everything we had done and asked us to visit him if ever at the hospital again. We grabbed a bite to eat and the medics took us back to the airport. We then flew back to our home base and restocked everything for the next mission before going home.

The Outcome:

An intra-aortic balloon pump and Swan-Ganz catheter were inserted several minutes after his admission. After placing the IABP, the hospital weaned off the dopamine, but by the next day his pressures had again declined. Unfortunately, even with the IABP, norepinephrine, and dobutamine, his cardiac function was not strong enough to perfuse his kidneys and they continued to fail. Several other medications were tried, but his blood pressure did not improve and he was placed on Extracorporeal Membrane Oxygenation (ECMO) two days after his arrival. This is a machine used to take over the work of the heart and/or the lungs. Unfortunately, his other organs had started to weaken by this time and he was not listed for a heart transplant.

Extracorporeal Membrane Oxygenation (ECMO)

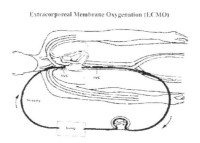

I transported another patient to this hospital by helicopter several days later and spoke with our patient. This was the first time I had spoken with a patient on ECMO. We talked for several minutes and he thanked me for my efforts. I remember him telling me he was "ready to go." After he said that, I remained quiet, not wanting to give him false hope because the likelihood of his long-term survival was extremely poor. A day or two after we spoke, he became short of breath and required a breathing tube. By this time, though, he had made it clear to his wife and healthcare givers that he wanted no other extreme lifesaving measures. After his family had gathered from around the country, his life support was withdrawn and he left this world peacefully with his family at his side.

Take Home Points:

For the Nurse or EMS Provider:

The primary reason this man was not listed for a heart transplant was because his organs were failing. I credit the sending hospital for transferring the patient, but maybe they waited too long. He was at this hospital for a week before he was transferred, and by that time his kidneys were failing. I sometimes wonder if the outcome might have been different had he been transferred sooner or if the sending hospital had taken more aggressive measures to improve his cardiac output. It's possible the outcome would have been the same, but the point I want to instill is the longer you wait to fix a problem, the worse it's going to get. If a patient has a low urine output (less than about 30 ml/hr.) or his creatinine is rising, the healthcare team needs to find the problem and fix it before irreversible damage is done. This is true for any abnormality.

Fluid is often given to increase blood pressure, but it's sometimes challenging in patients with heart failure. If the heart is weak and overstretched, the fluid you give might worsen the problem.

Remember Frank Starling's law and think of the heart similar to a rubber band. There is an optimal degree of stretch where the rubber band will snap back, or the heart contract most forcefully. If you overstretch either, however, you lose the optimal stretch and the force of recoil is diminished.

For the Public:

It's important to prevent and/or control coronary artery disease. Things you can do to limit the risk of heart attack include:

- Quit smoking - after 10-15 years of not smoking, your risk of death from heart disease is the same as if you had never smoked.
- Eat a heart-healthy diet.
- Exercise for at least 30 minutes on most days of the week. Talk to your doctor before starting an exercise program.
- Control your cholesterol and blood pressure.
- If you're at risk for heart disease, daily aspirin may reduce your chances of having a stroke or a heart attack. Talk with your doctor prior to starting aspirin treatment as aspirin has certain risks.
- Manage stress levels and get help for depression.

If you experience chest pain or other symptoms as discussed in the heart attack stories...please get these checked out ASAP. If a heart attack is corrected rapidly, there is a good chance of retaining cardiac function and living a healthy life. If you wait or ignore the pain, the pain might go away but the muscle can die and be replaced with scar tissue, ultimately leading to decreased function and a poor quality of life.

HEART ATTACK

Setting:

A 60 year old healthy man, who had never been to the hospital, experienced the worst chest pain of his life while home doing yard work. His wife called 911. Paramedics arrived within minutes, gave him aspirin, and took him to the nearest emergency department (ED). At the hospital, he became sleepy, still complaining of extreme and unrelenting chest pain. His heart rate was slow (in the 50s), but his blood pressure was normal. An electrocardiogram (ECG) was abnormal, with ST elevations in the inferior leads of the heart, II, III, and AVF. It became clear he was having a massive heart attack and would die without intervention. However, the necessary intervention was not available at this hospital and a helicopter was requested to transport him to one equipped to intervene. We fly patients with heart attacks routinely, but this would be a trip I'll never forget.

Everyday Language Of What Might Be Going On:

The electrocardiogram, sometimes called ECG or EKG, shows the electrical activity of the heart. This is the first test done when a patient comes to an emergency department with chest pain to help diagnose a heart attack. An abnormality on the ECG sometimes seen during an active heart attack is called ST elevation. A heart attack with this ECG abnormality is known as a STEMI, which stands for **ST** **E**levation **M**yocardial Infarction. This is a compelling signal of an active heart attack and suggests a part of the heart muscle is dying from not getting blood flow.

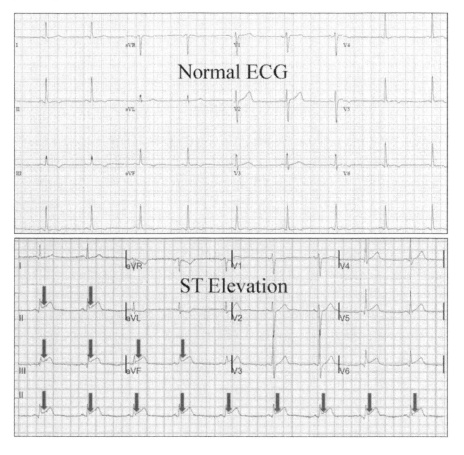

The definitive treatment for a heart attack is to open blood flow to the area of circulation that is blocked. Every minute is crucial once blood flow becomes obstructed. Most patients who die of a heart attack die within the first two hours of symptom onset. If the occlusion is opened quickly, patients often go home a few days later and live productive lives without residual effects. But, with each minute delay in opening the obstructed vessel, a greater portion of the heart muscle is likely to die. This leads to a decrease in normal heart function and increases the risk a patient will suffer or have serious complications, even death.

Blocked Artery   Healthy Artery

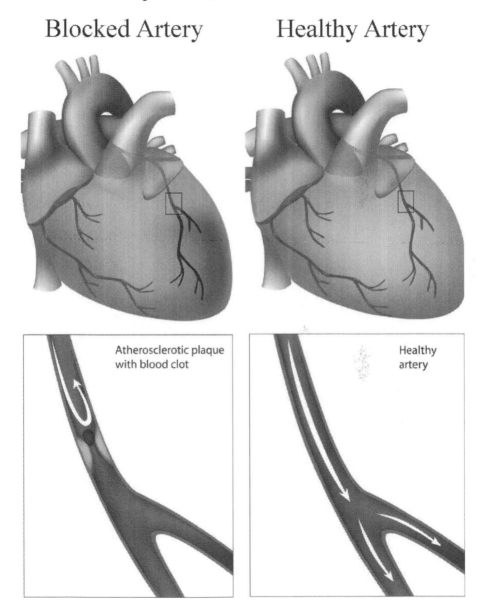

Atherosclerotic plaque with blood clot

Healthy artery

The two primary interventions to open blood flow are percutaneous coronary intervention (PCI) or by giving medications to break up the clot. If PCI can be done rapidly, it is the preferred method of treatment. PCI is performed by inserting a catheter through the skin in the groin or arm into an artery and opening the occlusion with a balloon, stent, or cutting device.

Both PCI and medications, however, have a time window in which they are effective. The treatment prior to opening the blockage is to try to minimize the size of the occlusion. This is why patients are encouraged to take aspirin immediately if they experience chest pain. Other medications given at the emergency department are used for the same reason, but work a bit differently to target several causes of blood clotting.

The Flight Out and Game Plan:

We had just finished restocking our equipment from an earlier flight when our pagers vibrated. I looked to see the message and read "Inferior STEMI, 60 year old male, elevation in II, III and AVF, HR in 50s". We were dispatched to the hospital with only that information and were airborne in minutes. The flight to the sending hospital took only 10 minutes. Based on the ECG pattern of reported ST elevation in leads II, III, and AVF, the heart attack was likely on the right side of the heart (inferior), which usually receives blood from the right coronary artery (RCA). The RCA also typically supplies the part of the heart that controls normal heart rate, known as the sinoatrial (SA) node.

These patients can drop their blood pressure quickly in response to nitroglycerin, which is a medication normally given to minimize chest pain in a heart attack. So if our patient had a low blood pressure, we would avoid this drug.

Even with a normal pressure, we would have to be careful giving it. Our goal was to make sure he had received aspirin and other blood thinners commonly given with STEMI and get him to the cardiac catheterization (cath) lab as fast as possible. Once at the cath lab, his occlusion could be ballooned open and a stent place.

The Transport:

Less than 20 minutes after being dispatched, we landed at a small community hospital and were escorted to the emergency department. The moment we walked in the hospital room we knew this was a life-threatening situation. On the bed in front of us lay an older gentleman, barely awake, and cool to the touch. His heart no longer pumped strong enough to adequately provide blood to his brain or extremities. He appeared drowsy but was aware enough to express he suffered from the worst chest pain in his life. His skin looked pale and his forehead glazed with perspiration. His heart rate was in the low 50s and his blood pressure had declined to 74/36. Most clinicians are worried when the systolic pressure (top number) is below 90 so 74 concerned us. If the pressure is too low, organs, including the heart, do not get blood flow. This creates further complications and can lead to death. Part of his heart already lacked blood flow. With a low blood pressure, his heart attack would only worsen and it became essential to increase his blood pressure.

The nurses were giving an intravenous (IV) fluid bolus at the maximum rate the pump could infuse, 999 ml/hr., and a nitroglycerine infusion was running. An infusion running at 999 ml/hr. is equal in volume to half a 2 liter of coke per hour. A fluid bolus is a volume of fluid intended to be given at a rapid rate and I thought to myself, *are you kidding?*

Administering a fluid bolus with an IV pump is a mistake I have, unfortunately, seen more than once. If a fluid bolus is what a patient needs to improve blood pressure, it needs to get in the body NOW, not over an hour. We shut off the nitroglycerine infusion and placed the IV fluid to a pressure bag. Pumps have limitations and by placing the IV bag in a pressurized device, the fluid travels into the body at a much faster rate.

Within minutes his blood pressure rose to an acceptable, 96/48, and he became a bit more awake. His heart rate, however, remained in the mid-50s. We placed him on our monitor, put temporary pacing pads on his chest and set them to start pacing if his heart rate went below 50. These pads are similar to an automated external defibrillator (AED). They stick to the body and are placed so the heart lies between two large pads and then connect to our patient monitor. Our monitor can then deliver an electrical impulse at a set rate with each impulse triggering the heart to beat. With these pacing pads on and set to fire, if his heart rate dropped suddenly, our monitor would immediately take over and trigger a heartbeat

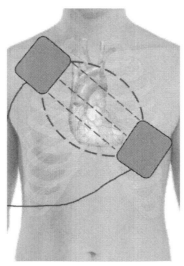

There are other methods, aside from pacing, available to help speed the heart rate. Atropine is a drug commonly given to increase heart rate, but we didn't want to give it quite yet. Although giving it might speed his rate, it might also cause the heart muscle, which was not getting blood flow, to work harder, ultimately causing more damage. He had been given the usual medications to help prevent further occlusion and placed on a 100% oxygen mask, called a non-rebreather. This was not likely helping the underlying problem because no matter how saturated the blood is with oxygen, if it can't get to the muscle tissue, it can't do much good. We continued this anyway, put him on our cot, and left the hospital, hoping to get to the cath lab before he crashed.

We loaded him in the helicopter, the pilots began their start up procedures, and the chaos began. Usually, the entire crew is communicating during takeoff for increased safety but we knew our patient needed our full attention so we asked the pilots to isolate us. This allowed my partner and I to communicate without hindering the pilots in their duties. Our destination was only a 5-minute flight, but it looked like our patient might not make it if we didn't do something.

We lifted for our destination and our patient became even sleepier. His heart rate was still in the 50s, but we couldn't get a blood pressure with our equipment. Fortunately, his pulse in his carotid and radial arteries were still able to be felt. This reassured us that no matter what our monitor read, his heart was pumping. On the monitor, his oxygen level began to decrease and his respirations suggested he needed a breathing tube placed. This is a plastic tube used to assist a patient in breathing. One end is placed into the trachea through the mouth. The other end is connected to either a ventilator or a breathing bag (ambu bag) for manual resuscitation. Placing a breathing tube can be dangerous, especially in the cabin of a helicopter. If this had been a long flight we would have done it without hesitation. However, since our destination was now only 4 minutes away, we would almost be on the ground by the time we had everything ready to place the tube.

The dilemma we faced was whether to try this in the air, in a position which lowered our chances of success, or wait 3 or 4 more minutes until we were on the ground. We decided to wait. We thought that if we could increase his heart rate, his brain might perfuse more and he'd wake up, so we gave atropine. After administering the drug, we watched the monitor for any increase in his heart rate but nothing happened. His rate remained in the 50's and he became more and more sleepy. Since we had already placed the pads and connected them to our monitor, we increased the pacing rate from 50 to 70. Our monitor then sensed his heart rate was too slow and delivered short bursts of electrical energy through defibrillation pads 70 times a minute. After each burst, the electricity travelled to his heart and it contracted. Before I knew it, we were on final approach to our destination. During landing, we arranged the equipment needed to place the tube and planned to place it as soon as we landed.

Although it was only another minute before we reached the ground, it seemed like an eternity. We landed, the pilots shut down the aircraft, and we put the patient in a position to place the breathing tube. We turned the cot and my partner placed the tube like he had done it a million times. This procedure still gets my heart racing, because the consequences of failure are so great. We then secured the tube and by this time, our monitor had gotten an acceptable blood pressure of 98/54. His heart began to beat above our set pacing rate and his condition looked a bit more stable. We used an ambu bag to manually breathe for the patient and followed the security escort to our destination.

The cardiac cath team was ready and waiting on us and we updated them on the course of events that transpired while in flight. Our patient had a pulse and a decent blood pressure but now needed help from a machine to breathe. Most of all, he needed the occlusion blocking blood flow to his heart opened. Whether he would live or die was beyond our control, but we had done everything in our power to improve his chances for a good outcome. We slowly walked to the helicopter, returned to base and made our aircraft ready for the next call.

The Outcome:

The patient had severe right coronary artery blockage which was opened and a stent placed. He had a full recovery and is enjoying a second chance at life.

Take Home Points:

For the Nurse or EMS Provider:

Aspirin is the first drug you should give to a patient with a heart attack...give this drug before you give oxygen. The underlying problem is that blood isn't getting to muscle and your goal is to prevent this from getting worse. No matter how saturated the hemoglobin is, if it's not getting to the tissue, it's useless.

Be careful giving nitroglycerin to patients with an inferior heart attack (ST elevation in leads II, III, AVF) because their blood pressure might drop significantly. Inferior infarctions are likely to involve the right ventricle, which then pumps blood to the lungs and then the left side of the heart. Even a small amount of nitroglycerin can dilate the entire venous system and the right side of the heart will no longer be able to move blood to the left. This is why, in addition to stopping the drug, you give fluid as rapidly as possible if blood pressure drops after giving these patients nitroglycerin.

If your goal is to give a fluid bolus quickly, don't put it on a pump, use a pressure bag and connect it to the largest IV you can (smallest gauge). A pump will take an hour to get one liter in the circulation.

No matter how many times you intubate or take part in an intubation, have several backup plans before you start. Although I didn't discuss this, we had in our bag a King Airway, an intubating bougie, and equipment for a surgical airway. We now carry a glidescope, which is an awesome piece of equipment to increase the likelihood for successful intubation.

For the Public:

Don't mess around with chest pain. Heart attacks can involve discomfort in the center of the chest that lasts more than a few minutes. It might go away and come back. Most patients describe the pain as either an uncomfortable pressure, squeezing, fullness or flat out pain. If you experience it, take an aspirin and get to the nearest emergency department.

Not everyone with a heart attack will feel chest pain. It has been reported that 42 percent of women and 31 percent of men never have chest pain.

Some people do not experience chest pain and not all signs of a heart attack are obvious so also look out for the following:

- Discomfort in other areas of the upper body such as pain or discomfort in one or both arms, the back, neck, jaw or stomach.
- Shortness of breath with or without chest discomfort.
- Breaking out in a cold sweat, fatigue, nausea or lightheadedness.

DOC...I THINK YOU'RE WRONG

Setting:

A 70 year old male with heart failure had stopped taking his diuretic medication. After missing two or three doses, he progressively became short of breath to the point he could not even walk a few steps without having to sit and rest. His granddaughter, who had been staying at his house, came home and found him in his chair unable to get up without becoming winded. She immediately recognized something was wrong and called 911. Paramedics came to the house within ten minutes and put him on their monitor. This showed his oxygen saturation to be well below normal and his heart rate and blood pressure both were significantly elevated. They placed him on a 100% oxygen mask, called a non-rebreather, and drove him to the closest emergency department (ED) while the granddaughter followed behind in her car.

The physician working at the emergency department had trouble obtaining an accurate history from the patient because he was too exhausted to even speak more than a few words. The physician spoke with the paramedics and granddaughter to help understand what might be going on, and then ordered several tests. After reviewing the lab results, chest x-ray and history, he diagnosed the patient with congestive heart failure exacerbation, ordered an intravenous (IV) diuretic, and started a nitroglycerin IV infusion.

The patient, even with a 100% oxygen non-rebreathing oxygen mask, continued to have difficulty breathing and his oxygen levels had not improved all that much. This emergency department was a freestanding ED, not connected to a hospital, and had limited resources, so he needed transferred to a higher level of care. The physician thought the medications he had given would improve the patient's symptoms, initiated transfer, and requested a helicopter for transport.

Everyday Language Of What Might Be Going On:

With decreased blood flow to the kidneys, several chemicals are released by the body signaling them to retain fluid. This is good in a normal person and helps to prevent dehydration and maintain blood pressure. A person in heart failure (HF), also called congestive heart failure (CHF), has a weak heart which cannot pump the same amount of blood as a normal heart. This may cause the kidneys to not receive normal blood flow and they attempt to compensate for this, similarly to dehydration, by retaining fluid.

The problem in HF, as in this case, is that the arteries and veins are already filled with fluid, it's just not getting to the kidneys. Because the weak heart cannot move this extra fluid, it accumulates and can eventually leak out of the vascular system and into other areas of the body. One example of this is the edema sometimes seen in ankles. As this condition progresses, the fluid eventually backs up into the pulmonary vasculature system and into the lungs. This fluid impairs gas exchange between the lungs and blood, causing shortness of breath. Diuretics are prescribed to prevent the fluid from accumulating and failure to take these medications can lead to fluid overload and pulmonary edema, as in this case.

Pulmonary Edema

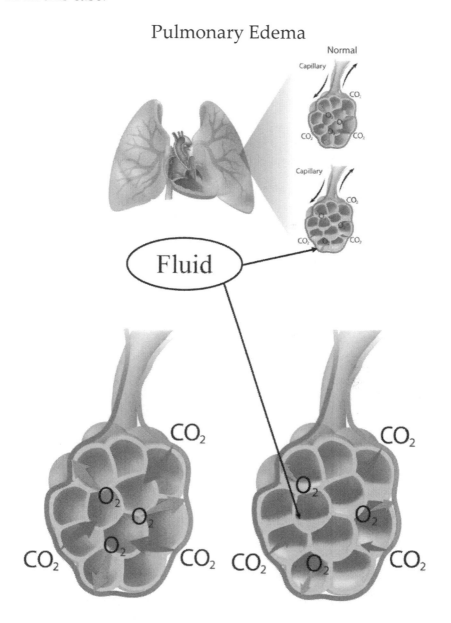

The Drive Out and Game Plan:

No aircraft could fly this day because of poor visibility, so we headed out in a mobile intensive care unit (MICU). By helicopter, this would be a 5-minute flight but by ground it would take almost half an hour. Ironically, we had left this same freestanding emergency department 3 hours prior, and as we left, saw paramedics bringing in a patient on a 100% non-rebreather oxygen mask. This would prove to be the same patient we had now been asked to transport. I telephoned the sending hospital while en route and spoke with our patient's nurse to get an update on his status. The underlying problem seemed clear: he was fluid overloaded. By treating this type of problem early, you can often avoid placing a breathing tube because the patient progressively improves as fluid is removed from his body.

The sending physician had given two important medications to improve the patient's condition: nitroglycerin and furosemide, also known as Lasix. Nitroglycerin dilates the vasculature system of the body. Giving this allowed for an increased space for fluid to accumulate and instead of overflowing into the lungs, fluid might remain in the vascular system. Nitroglycerin can also reduce the work load of the heart and allow it to pump more effectively. Lasix had been given to provoke an increased urine output from the kidneys.

Positive pressure ventilation, also known as CPAP or BiPAP, was a potential therapy this patient might benefit from. When positive pressure is applied to the lungs, excess fluid is pushed back into the vasculature system, allowing for better oxygenation. This machine can only be applied if the patient is awake enough to breathe with the machine and protect his airway. Unfortunately, it was not available at this particular emergency department. Regardless, it sounded as if this patient might not be awake enough to use either, even if they did have one.

We planned to increase the nitroglycerin as high as possible without dropping his blood pressure too low. If the foley catheter bag only had a minimal volume of urine, we would give another dose of Lasix. If he was awake enough, we planned to place him on our BiPAP machine.

The Transport:

We arrived at the emergency department and walked into the small eight bed unit to find an unresponsive patient on a 100% oxygen non-rebreather mask. He didn't open his eyes, even after repetitive yelling of his name and pinching his skin. He had a heart rate way above normal in the 140s and a high blood pressure of 192/86. The man could not adequately breathe and needed a breathing tube, so I asked the nurse if she'd get the attending physician while we put the patient on our monitor.

My partner increased his nitroglycerin IV infusion to lower his blood pressure and began to place a foley catheter to monitor his urine output while I spoke with the sending physician. I politely asked the doc if he'd help in placing a breathing tube to avoid doing this in the back of an ambulance. Sensing he wanted to avoid intubating our patient, he asked if we had a BiPAP machine. I told him yes, but asked if he thought that was best for the patient since he did not respond to any stimulation. With an annoyed face, he told us to just put him on our machine and said the patient would improve en route.

Unsatisfied with his answer and attempting to prove the need for a breathing tube with lab values, even though apparent simply by looking at the patient, I suggested we check an arterial blood gas (ABG). This helps determine gas exchange by measuring the acidity (pH) and levels of oxygen and carbon dioxide in the blood. An ABG would conclusively tell us if we needed to intubate by providing an actual oxygen or carbon dioxide (CO_2) level. A low oxygen or extremely elevated CO_2 level, as I suspected, would show he could not adequately breathe on his own. To my surprise, the doc said he preferred we just go and walked away.

This put us in a difficult and awkward situation. An emergency room physician, with all his training and education, should understand this machine is not intended to be used on unresponsive patients. Several thoughts went through my mind. *Do we go ahead with placing a breathing tube even after he asked us to go, or leave with an unresponsive patient, unable to protect his own airway?*

We wanted to provide the best treatment for our patient, but if things went bad with the intubation, what would we do? The doc had, after all, recommended we not intubate. I went ahead and put him on the BiPAP machine and turned the oxygen to 100%. But I did not think BiPAP would help our patient at this point. He was too sleepy to breathe with the machine and we were only delaying the inevitable.

His heart rate continued to stay elevated in the 140s and his blood pressure had only decreased modestly, so we again increased the nitroglycerin IV infusion. Since there was very little urine in the foley catheter bag, we doubled the dose of Lasix that had been given earlier, moved him to our cot, and left with an uncertain feeling about what might happen once in the ambulance.

We loaded our patient in the back of the ambulance and began the journey to the accepting hospital. I sat in my chair, stared at our patient, and knew transporting him in this condition was not right. I knew even before we left, but was somewhat apprehensive about placing a breathing tube because of the physician's attitude.

Our patient would still not respond to anything. We shouted his name and pinched his skin, but nothing happened. After a minute or two of driving and 30 minutes left ahead of us, I said to my partner "We can't bring him in like this". My partner agreed. We began to get everything ready to place a breathing tube and yelled to the driver to pull to the side of the road. The truck stopped. We sedated our patient even though he was already unresponsive and lowered the head of the cot. Our patient now laid lifeless, face up and flat on the cot, and we proceeded with the intubation.

Often when we intubate, we place a special mask over the nose and mouth, then breathe for the patient for a few minutes with an ambu bag and 100% oxygen. This allows us to fully saturate the blood with oxygen before attempting the procedure. We chose to avoid this with our patient. I had anticipated the likely need for the breathing tube at the emergency department by setting the BiPAP at 100% oxygen and to a level that was, in effect, acting like an ambu bag valve mask.

We gave the sedative about a minute to take effect in case he might have been aware of his surroundings. I inserted a laryngoscope into his mouth and manipulated it until I could see his vocal cords. Once I had a good view, I placed the breathing tube through them and into the trachea.

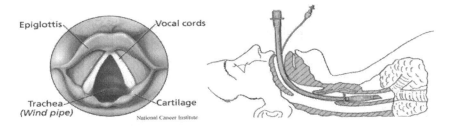

We confirmed it was in place, secured it, then placed him on our transport ventilator and attached a carbon dioxide (CO_2) monitor to continually measure the amount he exhaled. As we expected, the CO_2 measurements on our monitor were way above normal. He had been too sleepy to blow the carbon dioxide from his body which led to his altered mental status. A sigh of relief came over me after the intubation and I told the ambulance driver to continue to the accepting hospital.

The breathing tube was like placing a magic wand. His heart rate gradually lowered to normal, his blood pressure trended down to normal, and he looked much more comfortable. Over the course of the 30-minute transport, his CO_2 levels came down close to normal. Placing the tube and applying positive pressure to the lungs had forced the excess fluid out of his lungs and, about 5 minutes before we arrived at the accepting hospital, our patient began to waken.

This was a good sign and meant he was improving, but we didn't want him to wake up and inadvertently pull the breathing tube out, so we gave him a small dose of sedation. We took him to the intensive care unit and placed him in the bed while the nurses continued his nitroglycerin IV infusion and connected him to their ventilator and monitoring equipment. I spoke with the accepting physician and told him what had happened. He reaffirmed we had done the right thing and thanked us for our help.

The Outcome:

The patient continued to improve as fluid left his body. He received a few more doses of his diuretic and was extubated the next day. Two days later, he went home after receiving teaching about the importance of taking his blood pressure and diuretic medications to prevent this from happening again.

Take Home Points:

For the Nurse or EMS Provider:

Nitroglycerin helps reduce preload and afterload – this is often one of the first drugs ordered in patients with congestive heart failure exacerbation. By dilating the venous system, you provide a space for intravascular fluid to accumulate other than the lungs. By reducing preload and afterload, it allows the heart to increase output and helps get the diuretic to the kidney. It also helps dilate coronary arteries, providing more blood flow to the heart.

Initial dosing of Furosemide (Lasix) for patients in acute pulmonary edema[3]

- 0.5-1 mg/kg (40 mg) IV over 1-2 minutes / or dose equal to or 2.5 times greater than their maintenance dose
- May be increased to 80 mg if no adequate response in an hour
- Not to exceed 200 mg

BiPAP and CPAP are helpful for patients in congestive heart failure who present with signs of fluid overload. These cannot be used on unresponsive patients. Positive pressure applied to the lungs will help push excess fluid into the pulmonary vasculature and prevent further fluid from accumulating in the lungs.

For the Public:

This is another story that stresses the importance of taking your prescribed medications. This man stopped taking his diuretic and fluid accumulated in his lungs.

Patients with heart failure can experience shortness of breath when excess fluid builds up in the lungs. The heart can't keep up with all the fluid in the vasculature. Pay attention to ankle swelling, weight gain, shortness of breath, difficulty lying flat, fatigue, or persistent coughing, especially with white or pink tinged mucus. These may be symptoms of heart failure and need to be checked out by your doctor.

INTRACRANIAL HEMORRHAGE

Setting:

A 74 year old female with a history of hypertension met her son to eat one Saturday afternoon. Suddenly, midway through their lunch, the son noticed his mother speaking in a strange manner. Her speech became slurred, garbled, and barely comprehensible. When she tried to talk, only half of her face moved while the other half remained motionless. Not knowing what to do and thinking this might be a stroke, the son called 911. An ambulance arrived in less than five minutes and rushed her to the closest emergency department (ED). During the drive, however, the lady's symptoms had gotten much worse.

Movement on the right side of her body faded away and she became very sleepy. She faintly opened her eyes, but only after someone screamed in her ear. When asked her name, she mumbled words unrelated to the conversation. Suspecting a stroke, the physician at the emergency department sent her at once for Computerized Tomography (CT) imaging of the brain.

The scan showed a large amount of blood on the left side of her brain, confirming the diagnoses of hemorrhagic stroke. Unable to manage her condition at this hospital, the physician initiated transfer and requested a helicopter to transport the patient to the closest stroke center. In the 15 minutes it had taken to complete the CT scan, her mental status had continued to decline and her right arm and leg were now both completely flaccid. Out of nowhere, she began having a seizure, violently jerking and shaking her left arm and leg.

Everyday Language Of What Might Be Going On:

Anyone who experiences sudden numbness, tingling or weakness on one side of the body must consider stroke as the cause. Other symptoms of stroke might include vision changes, trouble speaking, sudden confusion, problems walking, or a severe sudden headache different from other headaches. Strokes are caused by altered blood flow to any part of the brain. This alters oxygen delivery to that area of the brain and it becomes injured. The longer it is without oxygen, the more brain cells die. Specific parts of the brain control specialized functions of the body, injury to these areas alters normal function, and this is where the physical abnormality is noticed. For example, as in this case, she bled on the left side, which controls right sided movements.

There are several ways in which a stroke might occur. 1) The most common is called an ischemic stroke, which is caused from obstruction, or clot, within a blood vessel supplying blood to the brain and happens in roughly 85% of cases. 2) A hemorrhagic stroke, as in this case, occurs when a weakened blood vessel ruptures and is most commonly caused by uncontrolled hypertension. 3) TIA's, or transient ischemic attacks, sometimes called "mini strokes," are caused by smaller blood clots that the body is able to break apart rapidly to restore blood flow. Healthcare professionals must know the nature of a stroke to guide treatment. This needs to be done quickly to improve outcomes. Also, procedures and medications to correct strokes are only helpful if provided within hours of symptom onset.

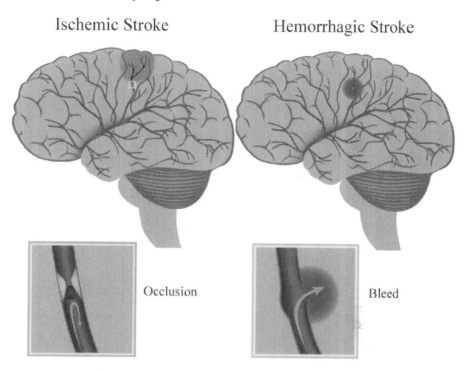

Ischemic Stroke   Hemorrhagic Stroke

Occlusion   Bleed

For an ischemic stroke (clot obstruction), the immediate goal, until corrective measures can be provided, is to allow for a higher than normal blood pressure. This allows for blood flow to the areas of the brain downstream of the occlusion. If treated promptly after symptom onset, a "clot-busting" medication can be given to some individuals to break up the obstruction. In certain hospitals, specialized physicians can use a wire to go into the arteries feeding the brain to remove or break up the clot, similar to PCI treatment for a heart attack.

This lady had a hemorrhagic stroke and was bleeding into her brain. The primary treatment for hemorrhagic stroke is to prevent further expansion of the bleed. If bleeding is not stopped, it grows and compresses more and more brain tissue, because the skull is ridged and cannot expand. With continued bleeding, symptoms progressively worsen. Even if the bleeding stops, the blood that has escaped from the vasculature can linger and hinder normal blood flow.

Healthcare workers try to prevent expansion by correcting bleeding disorders and preventing extreme elevations of blood pressure. The patient is transported as soon as possible to a center capable of either removing the blood/clot, or possibly even a part of the skull, to allow room for the excess volume of blood and fluid. In some parts of the brain, blood that comes into contact with brain tissue may trigger a seizure. This patient needed transferred to a center that had the ability to correct the bleeding and/or surgically remove excessive blood/clots from the cranium to relieve the excessive pressure from brain tissue.

The Flight Out and Game Plan:

The morning had been slow this day until around noon when my pager vibrated in my flight suit pocket. Our flight team met at the helicopter and was airborne within 8 minutes of the page. The hospital was almost 40 miles from our base which is a 15 minute flight. En route, we radioed for a patient update. Our patient was having a hemorrhagic stroke with a deteriorating mental status, and she had just begun to have a seizure. The game plan included stopping the seizure, keeping her blood pressure under control, and finding out if she took any blood thinners, such as Coumadin or aspirin. It was important to ask family if she had any disorders that might make her prone to bleeding so these could be corrected. It appeared as if she might need a breathing tube placed. Patients with deteriorating mental status often have trouble protecting their airway and breathing on their own. All of this needed to get done while still transporting her as fast as possible to an institution equipped to manage her problem. The sooner she could get there, the better her odds at full recovery.

Since she had seized, medications needed to be given, if not yet administered, to either stop or prevent this from occurring again. Seizures in mid-flight are dangerous for both the patient and the transport team. A jerking body in the back of a helicopter at 2,000 feet is not safe. The cabin windows are designed, in case of an emergency, to push out with only 40 lbs. of pressure. She had symptoms of an elevated intracranial pressure because of the increased volume (blood) in the skull. If her mental status was declining, we would give a medication called mannitol if it hadn't been given yet. Mannitol is a diuretic which helps remove fluid from the brain. Giving this would hopefully lower the pressures in her cranium and allow for more normal brain function, resulting in improved mental status.

The Transport:

We landed and followed security to the emergency department and walked into what might be described as a traffic jam, with hospital workers running about the ED. While we were en route, a full cardiac arrest came in to that same emergency department. Many hospital personnel were required to manage the patient in the other room, and ours had not been seen recently. We looked at our patient and she clearly needed our attention, but thankfully was no longer seizing. Lying in the bed was an unresponsive, almost lifeless, thin, elderly lady with minimal breathing movements. We needed to do several things as fast as possible before leaving. The hospital had placed two intravenous (IV) lines, but one had come out during the seizure, so my partner quickly placed another in her forearm. Certain drugs are not compatible in the same line and we needed the ability to administer several drugs simultaneously. Our next priority was to establish an airway without allowing her blood pressure to get too high.

While my partner drew up the intubation drugs, I hurried to place an arterial line. This is similar to an IV placed in the vein but sits in an artery and allowed us to better manage and monitor her blood pressure every second. Blood pressures obtained with a cuff take longer to get and are not as accurate as an arterial line. I quickly sterilized her wrist, placed a small needle into the radial artery and put a thin sterile wire through the needle into the artery. Then I removed the needle, leaving only the wire in the artery, and advanced a small sterile plastic catheter over the wire. I removed the wire, connected the catheter to our pressure monitoring device, and then secured the line with tape. Before I could dispose of the sharps I had used, our patient began to seize again. Afraid the arterial line would come out and begin to bleed profusely, I held her arm while my partner gave a drug called lorazepam (Ativan) that both stopped seizures and provided a desired sedating effect.

Within a minute after pushing the medication, her seizure stopped. This was our chance to place the breathing tube while she was still and motionless. Sometimes, the act of placing the tube can trigger spikes in blood pressure and worsen intracranial bleeding, so we gave several drugs to help prevent this. Once given, my partner opened her mouth, inserted a laryngoscope, manipulated the scope to view her vocal cords, and placed the tube into the trachea.

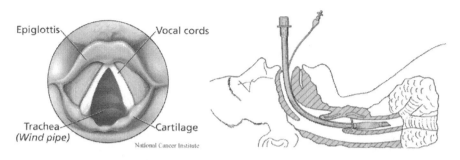

This went smooth except for one small detail. Her dentures became dislodged during the intubation. With the chaos we went through, I forgot to check for them. This was the least of our worries though and did not influence her care, so I removed them from her mouth, put them in a small bag, and continued working.

We confirmed the tube was in the right location and secured it with tape. Often after we intubate, if we expect the transport to be uncomplicated and if the flight isn't too long, one of us will manually ventilate the patient. We needed the extra hands, though, so we connected the breathing tube to our transport ventilator. Her blood pressure doubled the norm, now around 230/100. This was way too high and might further worsen her condition. We needed to give something to lower her blood pressure, relieve pressure on the brain, and prevent another seizure. I didn't want her to seize again in mid-flight, but it was imperative to get her blood pressure under control before we did anything else.

We started an intravenous infusion to lower her blood pressure, which began working almost instantaneously. Next, we gave the drug mannitol to relieve pressure on her brain,

125

caused from the bleeding. Then, we started another drug called phenytoin to prevent another seizure. With so many IV lines and tubes, everything resembled a bowl of spaghetti. It took several minutes to get organized and we then lifted her to our cot. After the move, she began to waken and reach for her breathing tube. I was unsure if the sedation was wearing off or the mannitol had started to work, but this was a good sign and suggested she at least had some neurological function. Regardless, the last thing we needed was the breathing tube out, so we gave another dose of the sedative we used to originally stop the seizure. Minutes later, she stopped reaching for the tube.

Thirty minutes after our arrival, with our patient now stabilized, we were ready to go. Our patient was sedated and had a secure airway. Her blood pressure was trending downward and she was no longer seizing. With the patient already on our cot, we secured the ventilator, monitor, and pumps to the cot then left the hospital. Once at the helicopter, we loaded her into the cabin, prepared to lift off, and gave one more dose of sedation. The flight to the accepting hospital proved to be uneventful. After a fourteen minute flight, we were almost home free and landed at the stroke center.

When possible, we try to unload with the aircraft running to save time, but there were too many IV lines, pumps, and other equipment to do this safely. The pilots powered off the helicopter and we carefully inched her from the helicopter and took her to the designated intensive care unit without any other incidents. She looked calm and peaceful as we finished the transport. We had reached our blood pressure goal, placed a breathing tube, an arterial line, another IV, treated the seizure, and brought her to an institution capable of managing her stroke.

The Outcome:

Several hours later, the patient went to the operating room and had a large blood clot removed from her cranium. This alleviated the excess pressure on her brain and allowed it to receive more normal blood flow. Although many brain cells had already died, some did recover and she was discharged several weeks later to a skilled nursing home with decreased function in her right arm and leg. It's unknown if she will ever be strong enough to walk again but her memory and mental function are normal.

Take Home Points:

For the Nurse or EMS Provider:

For patients with stroke symptoms, it's important to know the medications they normally take, especially if they take any blood thinners or antiplatelets (Coumadin, ASA, Plavix, etc.). This will impact whether the accepting hospital will give certain medications or blood products to reverse the effects of those medications.

One of the biggest potential pitfalls in treating stroke patients, with potentially major consequences, is to let their blood pressure get too low: if you do, their brain will not perfuse. It only takes minutes for brain cells to die from poor perfusion.

In general, ischemic strokes are allowed to become hypertensive and hemorrhagic strokes have more tightly controlled blood pressures.

While there is no clear evidence for blood pressure management with ICH, The American Heart Assoc. / American Stroke Assoc. ICH BP guidelines (2010) state that in patients presenting with a SBP of 150 to 220 mm Hg, acute lowering of SBP to 140 mm Hg is probably safe [4].

For the Public:

If you take the drug Coumadin, it's extremely important to take the proper dose, eat the right foods, and monitor your INR. Failing to do so can increase the likelihood of stroke.

Do not delay seeking treatment for a suspected stroke. Many therapies to correct these symptoms are not offered if too much time has elapsed from symptom onset. The longer you wait to get treatment, the more likely you'll have a poor outcome.

Symptoms of stroke commonly include sudden numbness, tingling, or weakness on one side of the body. Other symptoms might include vision changes, difficulty speaking, sudden confusion, problems walking, or a severe sudden headache different from other headaches.

TIAs or "mini strokes" need to be taken seriously and are often warning signs of an impending larger stroke.

DIABETIC KETOACIDOSIS

Setting:

This is a story about a 26 year old young diabetic woman, who was 14 weeks into her second pregnancy. She had been feeling ill and attributed this to prenatal sickness. Her family had noticed she began to use the bathroom every hour or two and seemed to always be drinking a large cup of water. She wouldn't eat her food and, except to use the restroom, just laid in bed complaining of abdominal pain and nausea. She quit taking her insulin because of her illness and, over the course of several days, grew more and more drowsy. This progressed until the next morning she became almost completely unresponsive and her family called 911. The ambulance came minutes later and took her to the closest emergency department (ED).

At the ED she remained nonverbal and barely opened her eyes, even to deep painful stimulation. Hospital staff would shout her name so loud it could be heard way down the hall. Her only response, however, was to gaze toward the yell and drift back to sleep. Concerned the patient's altered mental status might not allow her to adequately breathe, the emergency room physician placed a breathing tube minutes after her arrival. Blood and urine were both sent for testing, and she went for immediate brain imaging to rule out a stroke.

Her blood glucose levels came back ten times the normal limit at over 1000. She also had ketones in both her blood and urine. A test called an arterial blood gas (ABG) was obtained, which showed an extremely acidotic blood level. Her pH was only 6.9, a level almost incompatible with human life. Her potassium more than doubled the average, as demonstrated by ECG abnormalities which, if they continued, could cause death. Based on those test results, she was diagnosed with diabetic ketoacidosis (DKA) and hyperkalemia. Further tests also suggested a possible pneumonia, with a white blood cell count three times the norm, and an abnormal chest x-ray.

In light of her pregnancy, the emergency room doctor decided to transfer her to a medical center better equipped to manage her critical condition and requested a helicopter for transport. While waiting for the aircraft, the sending physician began treatment measures, including a calcium intravenous (IV) infusion to prevent cardiac arrest from her high potassium, insulin to help shift glucose into cells, and an antibiotic to treat presumed pneumonia. She was also given four liters of IV fluid over several hours because she was likely extremely dehydrated.

Everyday Language Of What Might Be Going On:

Human cells need glucose (sugar) to function. Insulin facilitates the movement of these molecules from the blood into cells. Diabetics either do not make insulin (type I), or their cells do not respond properly to it (type II), leading to a higher amount of glucose in the blood and not enough in the cells. Medications, including insulin, are prescribed to diabetics to enable movement of glucose from the blood into cells. Failure to take prescribed medications can result in not enough glucose for the cell and too much in the blood, creating a cascade of problems.

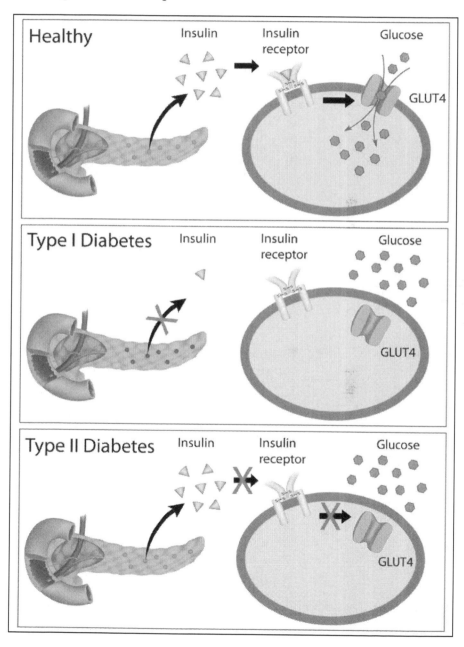

With glucose accumulation in the bloodstream, glucose molecules act to hold water in the bloodstream, and eventually this water passes through the kidney and leaves the body as urine. This causes an excessive urine output leading to dehydration. As water is also pulled from the cells they become dehydrated and signals are sent to the brain triggering a feeling of thirst. Dehydration and high blood sugar can cause fatigue, weakness, nausea, vomiting, confusion, and eventually may lead to coma.

Ketoacidosis is a complication sometimes seen in type I diabetics. These patients cannot make insulin, and without it, no glucose is carried into cells. This triggers a series of hormonal responses, causing the body to break down fat into the form of fatty acids for metabolism. The end products of these acids are known as ketones. As cells continue to be deprived of glucose, more fatty acids are made, resulting in a more acidotic blood level than normal. The body then attempts to compensate for the acidotic environment by increasing the respiratory rate and blowing off carbon dioxide (CO_2). In an acidotic environment, the potassium normally in the cells enters the blood and the level in the blood rises, as seen in this case. It's important to note that although blood levels can be elevated, total body potassium is often depleted as potassium leaves the body with excessive urine output.

Immediate treatment is focused on replenishing the lost fluid, monitoring and normalizing potassium, and monitoring blood pH levels. Correcting the ketoacidosis involves giving insulin to move glucose and potassium into the cells and out of the bloodstream. This will usually resolve symptoms if treated promptly. But, if ketoacidosis is severe enough to cause an extremely high potassium level or acidosis with a pH below 6.9 or 7.0, calcium and bicarbonate are sometimes given to prevent complications such as cardiac arrest.

The Drive Out and Game Plan:

This day, as a result of poor weather conditions, it was only intermittently flyable, and our first flight request had been turned down because of inclement weather. We had just finished the prior mission by ambulance and were on our way back to base when our pagers vibrated and read…"26 year old female, 14 weeks pregnant, DKA with pH 6.9, potassium 9.4, glucose > 1000, intubated on 2 drips." I looked at my partner and both of our hearts sunk. Two lives depended on us, one of them not even born, and I yelled to our driver to drive "hot". We headed to the sending hospital with lights and sirens running. If weather permitted, the helicopter would meet us at the hospital's helipad. Unfortunately, this flight too was declined, forcing us to complete the trip with our mobile intensive care unit. We arrived there about 15 minutes later but had an hour drive to the accepting medical center, even with lights and sirens.

Few details had been relayed to us regarding her current status, but she sounded to be quite sick. A pH of 6.9, if not corrected rapidly, can result in death. Since this was a young woman with a 14-week fetus, we were concerned for both the patient and her unborn child and wanted to do everything possible to improve their chances of survival. Cases like this make you sit back and think about the importance of life and loved ones. Since we knew this was diabetic ketoacidosis; our two primary goals focused on ensuring adequate fluid had been given and attempting to get her glucose trending down towards normal. We planned to review the most recent labs, specifically her blood glucose and arterial blood gas, and be as quick as possible to move her to a higher level of care. Having been at that unit for several hours, we expected her condition to be improving, but this would prove to not be the case.

The Transport:

We parked our ambulance in front of the emergency department, unloaded our equipment, and walked in. The inside of the ED looked like a crowded parking lot. Beds with patients in them lined the hallway while the nurses ran around trying to take care of them all. The secretary pointed us to our patient's room and we walked in. The nurse who had been taking care of her gave us a brief report and although our patient looked stable on the outside, internally she was getting much worse.

She had been given several liters of fluid through an intravascular (IV) infusion and her vital signs were normal with a heart rate in the high 90s and a blood pressure of 112/68. A breathing tube had been placed to secure her airway and a central line had been placed for larger and more stable venous access. She was breathing much faster than the set rate of the ventilator, subconsciously attempting to correct her acidotic state. To my surprise, however, she had not yet been placed on an insulin IV infusion and no labs had been drawn for over two hours.

Diabetics like this patient often require 30 to 60 units of insulin daily. She had only gotten 10 units over the past 3 or 4 days. Our patient was not going to improve without more insulin. Although the fluid she had gotten might help dilute the concentration of glucose, without insulin to move it into the cells she would continue to create fatty acids and ketones. I asked the nurse if we could have some to give our patient in transport since this is one of the few medications not supplied in our transport bags. The nurse said she had to get it from pharmacy, which might be a while. Unsatisfied with that answer, I politely asked if we could take some from the emergency department and mix up our own IV infusion. In a more firm tone, she restated that all insulin infusions must come from pharmacy and she would try to get it. While the nurse worked at obtaining the medication, we continued the calcium infusion they had started to prevent potential cardiac arrhythmias, as well as the IV fluid infusion that was correcting her dehydrated state. We placed her on our transport equipment, moved her to our cot, and were ready to go after 5 or 10 minutes.

The triggering cause of all our patient's serious problems stemmed from not having insulin in her bloodstream, so I asked again if we could have some before we left. We had another hour drive and I did not want our patient to wait that long before receiving it. Unfortunately for our patient, it was against policy for the emergency room to provide this particular drug to us and I was told it would still be "a while" and that pharmacy was working on it. Trying to not express my frustration I asked, "How long is a while" and she said it could be 30 minutes or more. Displeased with the situation and not knowing if we'd ever get the insulin, we left the bedside with our patient and walked outside. The weather, still poor with low visibility and rain, had not improved, and I regretted the fact we were not loading our patient into a helicopter. Nevertheless, we loaded her in the squad and began our journey to the accepting hospital.

The ambulance began to move and we checked a finger stick glucose which read high. Most glucometer machines, including ours, will only read "high" if a blood sugar is over

600. We reasoned that since she had only been given 10 units of insulin, her cells were not getting any glucose, she was still likely creating fatty acids for metabolism and her blood was probably still extremely acidotic. She still breathed very rapidly, attempting to correct her acidotic state, triggering the ventilator with each breath. The body can only compensate to a certain degree, however, and if her pH became low enough, it would eventually not be compatible with life.

While speeding down the highway with sirens screaming, we did all we could with the resources available to us to improve her current situation. We placed an arterial line in her wrist to monitor her blood pressure more accurately and continuously. Once this was in place, we rechecked her arterial blood gas to have a more definitive understanding of her condition. Specifically, we needed to know her pH and not allow it to become excessively low, which might lead to further shock or death.

It took a few minutes to collect the blood and run the test. Her arterial blood gas had not improved, and in fact, had only worsened. Her pH, already critically low (6.9) several hours ago, should have been increasing with treatment, had now dropped to 6.7. A normal pH is 7.4; most clinicians are concerned with a pH lower than 7.2. She was near a level incompatible with life. We gave two ampules of sodium bicarbonate, which might act as a buffer of the acid to raise her pH, buying additional time until insulin could be administered. No matter what we did, though, we were not going to correct the underlying problem without insulin.

We arrived at the accepting hospital in about an hour, hurried to her designated unit, and placed her in the assigned bed. The nurses connected our patient to the hospital ventilator and their monitoring equipment, and the accepting physician walked in. I gave the entire team the story. I expected them to question why she had not yet been started on an insulin IV infusion, so explained to them my multiple efforts and unsuccessful attempts at obtaining it. Still personally concerned about her pH level, I asked if I would be allowed to check one final arterial blood gas before I left, having brought the machine needed to do this with us to the bedside. Wanting to know the information himself, the physician said of course. We ran one final test and the pH had improved to 7.05. Although not even close to normal, and still very concerning, the bicarbonate had temporarily improved her acidotic state and she would soon have the drug she truly needed, insulin.

The Outcome:

She was placed on an insulin infusion not long after we left and her diabetic ketoacidosis resolved by the next day. Unfortunately, her hospital course was quite complicated. She had a severe pneumonia which took over her lungs. She spent several weeks on the ventilator, required a tracheostomy, and was even placed on Extracorporeal Membrane Oxygenation (ECMO) for a brief period. Sadly, the fetus did not survive but our patient made a full recovery and walked out of the hospital two months later.

Take Home Points:

For the Nurse or EMS Provider:

Patients in diabetic ketoacidosis (DKA) or hyperglycemic hyperosmolar non-ketotic syndrome (HHNS) are severely dehydrated. Expect initial fluids to be 0.9% normal saline run fairly quickly (15-20 mL/kg/hr.) for the first few hours followed by 0.45% saline (4-14 mL/kg/hr.) if serum sodium is normal or elevated; 0.9% NS is continued if hyponatremia is present. Dextrose is added when serum glucose reaches 200 mg/dL in DKA or 250-300 mg/dL in HHS[5].

The patient needed insulin and without it, she wasn't going to get better. When insulin is ordered for DKA, you need to make it a priority to get this ASAP but make sure you know the potassium level before you give it.

The potassium level rises in acidosis. As the number of hydrogen ions increase in the blood, these hydrogen ions move into the cell in exchange for potassium. This potassium is then lost via the kidney so total body potassium may be low even if it appears normal or high. With the administration of insulin and as the acidosis is corrected, the potassium will move back in the cell.

This is why potassium is monitored closely in DKA and typically given, even when normal. If the potassium falls too low (<3.3), insulin is usually held to prevent further movement into the cells[5]. If you don't replace the potassium, as it moves back into the cells, life-threatening arrhythmias may result.

Bicarbonate therapy is typically not used unless the pH is less than 6.9[5].

For the Public:

For diabetics, it's extremely important to take your insulin or other diabetic medications as prescribed and not skip doses. Keep track of your blood sugars and if they are continually high or low, go see your doctor.

High blood sugars are linked to many other diseases, such as coronary artery disease, strokes, hypertension, neuropathy, and kidney disease.

Severely elevated glucose levels can result in a medical emergency like diabetic ketoacidosis (DKA) or hyperglycemic hyperosmolar non-ketotic syndrome (HHNS). Both can lead to profound dehydration.

SHE'S BARELY BREATHING

Setting:

A 38 year old female developed persistent abdominal pain and, over the course of a week, became fatigued and drowsy. One morning, she woke up confused and too weak to even get out of bed. Unsure what to do, her husband called 911 and an ambulance took her to the closest hospital.

Upon arrival to the hospital emergency department (ED), she had further deteriorated, now minimally responsive with a rapid heart rate in the 130s. She was incontinent of stool, which looked to have a purplish-red tinged color. The attending physician sent her for brain imaging then ordered stool and blood testing to help find the cause of her altered mental status. While she went for imaging, the physician further questioned her husband to see if she had any past medical problems. Apparently, she had gastric bypass surgery several years prior to this event and subsequently developed persistent abdominal pain. She had been taking high doses of ibuprofen for several months because her pain worsened and she had several bloody bowel movements the past week.

The radiologist read her brain image but found no abnormalities. Lab tests showed below normal blood levels and her stool tested positive for having blood in it. Most women her age have a hemoglobin range anywhere from 12 to 15, hers was only 9. The physician diagnosed her with a gastrointestinal (GI) bleed although her symptoms did not correlate with her lab results. Sometimes, GI bleeding can lead to a high ammonia level, which might cause these kinds of symptoms. But this test had come back normal, leaving no clear reason why she was so sleepy. The physician did not get one important detail about her history, nor did he order one particular test that might have diagnosed the problem. This would not be apparent until at the accepting hospital.

Since the smaller rural hospital did not have the resources needed to find the bleeding source or the cause of her altered mental status, the physician initiated transfer to a higher level of care. He also ordered two units of packed red blood cells and requested a helicopter for rapid transfer to the hospital where she originally underwent bypass surgery.

Everyday Language Of What Might Be Going On:

This patient's bloody stool and low hemoglobin are likely the result of gastrointestinal bleeding, also called a GI Bleed. It's important for health care professionals to find the source and/or cause of GI bleeding. This is usually done with either upper GI endoscopy or colonoscopy, using a tiny camera attached to a long, thin flexible tube to visualize the GI tract.

An endoscopy inserts at the mouth to visualize the upper GI tract, including the esophagus, stomach, and the first part of the small intestine, called the duodenum. A colonoscopy inserts at the anus and allows visualization of the

144

lower GI tract, including the majority of the small intestine and the large intestine (rectum and colon). In upper GI bleeds, blood moves through the GI tract and mixes with intestinal contents to form dark, tarry colored stool. Conversely, blood that originates from the lower in the GI tract exits the body faster. There is less time for mixing of gastric contents, thus, stool appears more bright red and bloody. A bleeding source thought to be lower in the GI tract (bright red stool) often requires a colonoscopy to visualize the source, whereas, if thought to be higher (dark tarry stool / coughing blood), an upper GI endoscopy is the preferred test.

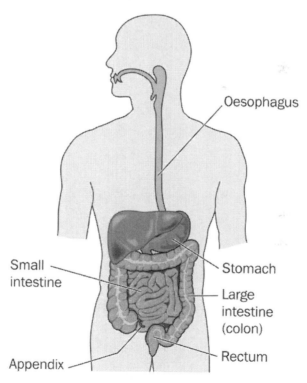

Ibuprofen (Advil, Motrin) is a nonsteroidal anti-inflammatory drug (NSAID) used to reduce fever and treat pain. It's intended to reduce inflammatory pain caused by conditions such as headache, back pain, arthritis, menstrual cramps, or small injuries. But ibuprofen has been known to increase the risk of serious GI bleeding. With severe GI bleeding and large losses of blood volume, the body tries to compensate for inadequate perfusion (blood flow) by increasing the heart rate, as in this case. If the bleeding is not corrected and intravascular volume replaced, blood pressure will fall as more and more blood is lost.

This patient's altered mental status was concerning and the cause was unclear. Sometimes GI bleeding can lead to altered mental states, but her ammonia level was normal. Should hemoglobin (blood) be present in the GI tract, some of it gets digested and absorbed, ultimately leading to the production of ammonia. Ammonia can cause a decrease in alertness and cognitive function. It's important to note that there may be many potential causes of her altered mental status. We simply did not know why at the time, and further studies needed to be done at the accepting hospital to find out. Clues to potential causes of many diseases are often discovered by obtaining a detailed patient history and physical exam. This is one of the most important diagnostic tools available to medical professionals, and in this case, a crucial piece of the puzzle was not relayed to the physician.

The Flight Out and Game Plan:

Thirty minutes before the end of my shift, my pager vibrated in the front chest pocket of my flight suit. I had been looking forward to several days off in a row, but with this flight, my mini-vacation would be on hold for several hours. The hospital requesting our services was roughly a 20-minute flight from our base and another 30 minutes to the accepting facility. If everything went perfect with the transport, which they seldom do, I would go home almost two hours late.

Almost an hour before this request, our pilots declined to take a flight because of stormy weather and poor visibility. The conditions had not improved much and we thought they might turn this one down as well. Our pilots assessed the radar, looked over the forecast, and said we could give it a shot but might have to abort the mission if we flew into poor weather.

Based on the patient report given to us by our dispatch center, it looked as if this might be a routine transport. Dispatch advised us our patient had a lower GI bleed with stable vital signs and a normal blood pressure. Her hemoglobin level was 9, and she received two units of packed red blood cells. Many times, physicians won't give blood unless the hemoglobin is below 7 or 8. Unless she had a major bleed, we thought her hemoglobin should be stable for the transport. Her heart rate had trended down to the 110s from the 130s before the blood transfusion. Even though still above normal, this indicated her intravascular volume status had improved. She needed minimal oxygen, 2 liters nasal cannula, and transports with patients on a nasal cannula are usually straightforward. I must admit that based on the report, this patient did not sound as if she needed urgent transport and I did not want to go on the flight.

Although sometimes inconvenient, getting out late on occasion is part of the job, so we jumped in the helicopter and lifted for our destination. I radioed for a patient update on the flight out but dispatch had no new information. The weather held and we landed at the hospital 20 minutes later. We would soon find out that one important detail about our patient had not been relayed to us: the degree to which her mental status was altered.

The Transport:

Once on the ground, our pilots advised us poor weather was moving our way. They estimated that in about an hour, conditions would not permit us to fly and they did not have enough duty time to wait for the weather to clear. This meant our pilots would have to leave without us if we were not ready to go in about 45 minutes. We would then be forced to either wait for the night duty pilots to return with an aircraft, or transport the patient via ambulance. Traveling by ambulance meant over a 90-minute drive to the accepting hospital. By this time, we should have already been getting off shift, and we dreaded a long ground transport. We told the pilots it should not take long and followed the security guard to the emergency department.

I walked in the room and, just by looking at our patient, knew the situation was not good. Her condition was much worse than we had been told and she might not survive such a long drive. We needed to fly her. She was completely unresponsive, with a heart rate now in the 150s. I thought her bleeding may have been worse than anyone expected. There was one reassuring sign, however; she still had a decent blood pressure, but this might drop if we didn't do something. We needed to do two things before attempting to transport her: start an intravenous (IV) fluid bolus to fill her intravascular space, and place a breathing tube. A fluid bolus is a large volume of IV fluid given at a rapid rate and might help lower her heart rate. Since she was too unresponsive to adequately breathe on her own, the breathing tube would allow us to breathe for her.

We applied a 100% non-rebreathing oxygen mask to allow for maximal oxygenation while we prepared to intubate.

My partner gathered the equipment and drew up the drugs needed for the intubation while I placed two more IVs. One of the IVs they had placed no longer worked and the other was too small to effectively administer large volumes of IV fluid. Next, we hung a liter bag of IV fluid, connected it to the biggest IV I had placed, and put this in a pressure bag to speed the rate of fluid delivery. She was likely intra-vascularly dry, and intubation drugs could cause her blood pressure to plummet. We wanted fluid "in the pipes", especially before placing the breathing tube. This also gave us an IV line with rapidly flowing fluid in which to push medications. Once injected into the line, they would flow into her body within seconds.

Next, I went and spoke with the attending emergency room physician and expressed my concerns for the transport. He appeared somewhat bothered, but I think it had been quite some time since he last assessed the patient. Emergency room doctors often are forced to see multiple patients, especially when working alone in a rural emergency department. They count on nurses to keep them informed of patient status changes. I'm not sure why he was not aware of her condition but, as I often say about a situation, *it is what it is*. There was no point in arguing about why; we just needed to fix it. Once the doc walked in, he realized the need for intubation and wanted to be the one who placed the breathing tube. He knew she needed one and perhaps felt obligated to place it.

The satisfaction of placing a breathing tube is difficult to describe. It's scary yet exhilarating at the same time. Once you push the drugs needed to place the tube, the patient's life is completely in your hands. But as soon as the tube passes through the vocal cords into the trachea, you feel a great sense of accomplishment and relief. Because of the devastating potential consequences of failure to intubate, it's crucial to keep up with this skill.

Although I wanted to place the tube, I appreciated the fact that this was his emergency room. The doc moved to the head of the bed and positioned her for intubation. We pushed drugs to both sedate, and then paralyze her, and she went into a deep sleep. The doc placed the breathing tube, we confirmed it was in the correct location, and we connected her to the hospital ventilator. I noticed one of our pilots had come to the room and could tell by the look on his face we had to go now. The only words he said were "weather is moving in" and I said "we're ready."

We moved her to our transport cot, and by this time she began to look more stable. Her heart rate trended down to the low 110s and she just appeared to be much more comfortable, like in a pleasant dream. Once secured to our cot and with our equipment in the proper place, we disconnected the hospital ventilator and took control of her ventilation. We left the bedside, manually breathing for the patient with an ambu bag. As we left, one of her sisters came up to me and expressed how grateful she was we had spoken with the emergency room physician about placing the breathing tube. She told me she knew her sister was much more comfortable now. This gave me a sense of pride and pleasure and I told her we would take good care of her sister.

Our patient loaded into the aircraft cabin without a problem. The pilots went through their normal startup checklists while we put the patient on our ventilator and secured everything for takeoff. I glanced out the helicopter window and noticed her family standing in the parking lot waiting for us to fly away. We lifted with an anticipated 30 minute flight to the accepting hospital. Although we had plenty of time to fly to there, we were uncertain if there would be enough time to fly home to base after the transport. Pilots are required by law to be on the ground 14 hours after their shift begins. This meant we had less than 80 minutes to fly to the hospital, drop off our patient, fly for fuel, and then return to base. This was going to be close and my mini-vacation might really be on delay now.

The rest of the flight was normal and routine. Most of the work had been done in the emergency room. She woke up slightly just before landing, so we gave her a small dose of a sedative drug which put her back into a deep sleep. We landed and unloaded the patient "hot", slang for with the aircraft running. While the pilots powered-down the helicopter, we took the patient to the intensive care unit and updated the accepting team about events necessitating a breathing tube. With the help of the hospital staff, we placed our patient on their bed. The nurses hooked up their monitoring equipment while we took ours off and the respiratory therapist connected her to the hospital ventilator.

We radioed to the pilots to begin start-up and informed them we would load "hot". After our patient was on the hospital monitor and we finished giving report, we began to briskly walk back to the aircraft. It was now almost 8 o'clock, 1.5 hours past our scheduled time off but still not home, and if we did not hurry, we would be stuck. We still had a 5-minute flight to the airport for fuel and another 10 minutes back to our base, leaving only 15 minutes for the pilots to fuel the aircraft.

We loaded "hot" and flew to the airport for fuel. As the fuel truck moved close to the helicopter, so did the weather.

The rain poured and the visibility dropped, and it was now too dangerous to fly. Even if the weather improved in 15 minutes, the pilots could not legally fly back to base. We gave it a few minutes, but the weather didn't get any better, forcing us to call a taxi and leave the aircraft at the airport for the next duty crew. At about 9:30 pm we finally got back to base and finished the paperwork for the transport. I was thankful to have a couple days off, even if delayed by 3 hours.

The Outcome:

There was no identifiable source of the rectal bleeding and it resolved spontaneously. Perhaps she took too much ibuprofen and this caused the bleed. Our patient had an overdose of a narcotic from an implanted pain pump that none of us knew she had. She had a history of chronic abdominal pain and the pump was placed to control her pain several months before this episode. Although she did have a GI bleed, it was the narcotic overdose that had caused her altered mental status. This is why none of the lab values made sense. The narcotic was held and dosing later decreased. As the narcotic wore off, she woke up, was extubated, and later discharged home.

A urine toxicology test, which would have identified the narcotic, was not done at the sending hospital. If we had a better history, or maybe examined her more closely, we may have considered narcotic overdose as a potential cause of her altered mental status. We overlooked this because of the condition she was in at the time and the need for prompt intubation. There are drugs that could have reversed the effects of the narcotic and she may have awakened.

Take Home Points:

For the Nurse or EMS Provider:

The best diagnostic tool is the history and physical exam. If any of us had investigated her history closer, we might have identified the pain pump, and possibly reversed the altered mental status with Narcan.

Naloxone (Narcan) reverses narcotic overdose.

Flumazenil (Romazicon) reverses benzodiazepine overdose.

Both can induce seizures, especially flumazenil and if the patient is dependent on narcotics or benzodiazepines.

For the Public:

Take the warnings on medication labels seriously and only take the prescribed dose. For many medications, only an extra pill or two is enough to cause serious complications.

Although questions by your healthcare provider may be frustrating to answer, it's important to answer them as completely as possible. These are invaluable in diagnosing medical conditions.

NSAIDs can increase the risk of gastrointestinal bleeding, ulceration, and perforation of the stomach or intestines. These events may be fatal and can occur at any time during use, even without warning symptoms. The elderly are at greater risk for serious gastrointestinal events.

UNEXPECTED CARDIAC ARREST

Setting:

When working a shift on the mobile intensive care unit (MICU), you can often expect more of a laid-back day as compared to helicopter transport. Patients requiring higher levels of critical care are typically transported by air unless the weather is poor. So on this beautiful summer day, I thought my shift would be slow and routine. As you'll soon find out, this would not be the case.

A chronically ill 68 year old man, who lived in a skilled nursing home, was taken to the emergency room after complaining of increasing shortness of breath. An electrocardiogram (ECG) and several other blood tests suggested he might have had a heart attack. However, there was no indication for emergent treatment since nothing suggested this was an acute heart attack, and cardiac catheterization was delayed.

Cardiac catheterization could not be done at this hospital and arrangements had been made for transfer to an institution with these capabilities. At the time of dispatch, the patient was stable and the sending physician requested ground transport via a mobile intensive care unit. After making the call to transfer the patient, he began to deteriorate, and little was done to improve his condition before we arrived.

Everyday Language Of What Might Be Going On:

Heart attacks can be diagnosed with either an electrocardiogram, better known as an ECG or EKG, or with certain blood tests. An ECG is a standard test done to assess the electrical activity of the heart. It can show signs of an ongoing or prior heart attack. One of the great benefits of the ECG is that abnormalities indicating an ongoing heart attack can be seen on the ECG hours before blood tests can detect it. This allows medical professionals to diagnose many heart attacks sooner.

The earlier a heart attack is diagnosed, the more likely medical professionals will be able to intervene and fix the underlying problem, before heart muscle cells die. Not all heart attacks can be diagnosed with an ECG, though, because sometimes abnormalities are either never present or not recorded. It's important to mention that ECG abnormalities that might be seen in an ongoing heart attack will fade away over the course of the several hours after the heart attack begins. These abnormalities are often not recorded because of time delays in reaching the hospital. When a heart attack is suspected, but ECG abnormalities are not clear, blood tests can be done to help diagnose a heart attack. Unfortunately, it takes longer for these blood tests to reveal a heart attack.

Heart muscle cells contain certain proteins to carry out normal functions. When these cells die or are injured, proteins are released into the bloodstream and can be detected by blood tests such as troponin, CK or CK–MB, and serum myoglobin. These proteins are not always detectable until several hours after a heart attack. This is why blood tests to detect a heart attack are done several times at various time intervals.

The cardiac catheterization lab, also called the cath lab, is special room in which coronary angiography is performed. This is a test that uses a tiny, flexible tube to inject dye into the bloodstream of the coronary arteries. Any obstructions or occlusions of blood flow can then be spotted with x-ray and treated by inflating a small balloon located at the end of the catheter.

Once the occlusion has been opened, stents can be placed to make sure the occluded area remains patent. The cath lab is not activated emergently for every heart attack that presents to an emergency department. If cardiac muscle cells have been without blood flow for a long time, those cells are not as likely to benefit as cells in which this happens suddenly. This is why only patients likely to benefit from prompt intervention are taken there right away.

This patient's ECG did not show he was having an ongoing heart attack; however, blood tests suggested he may have earlier because of elevations in the proteins mentioned previously. He didn't fit the criteria for emergent cath and was transferred to have a cath at a later date. It's possible this man's heart attack happened many hours before he came to the hospital and the acute changes sometimes seen on the ECG had gone away.

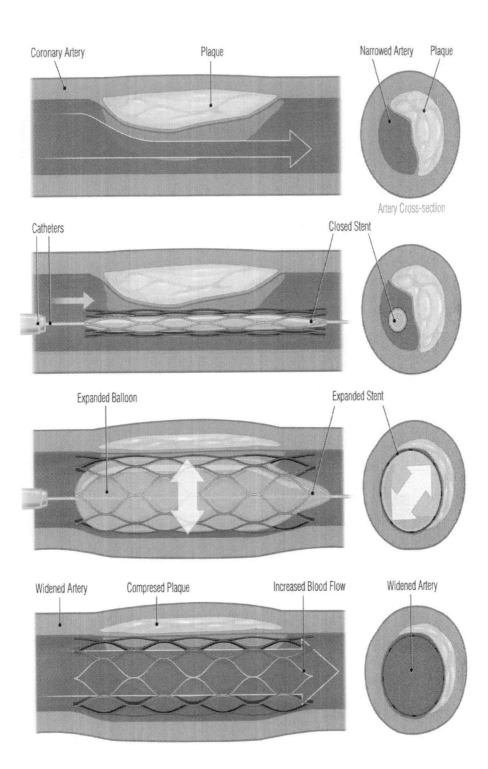

158

The Drive Out and Game Plan:

Patients that need urgent treatment or are unstable are typically transported by helicopter to avoid long time periods out of the hospital and/or to offer prompt intervention. So when working on the mobile intensive care unit, the adrenaline rush is not there like on the helicopter, unless the weather is poor. This day was sunny, and 99% of ground transports on a sunny day are routine and uneventful, so why would I expect anything different from this transport?

At around 9:00 AM, we headed out for a routine transfer from an emergency department at a rural hospital to the cardiovascular unit of a large teaching medical center. The patient would undergo cardiac catheterization within the next few days. Medications to treat a non-acute heart attack had been given, and he required just one intravenous (IV) infusion called heparin. This is a common medication given after a heart attack is suspected to prevent blood clots, potentially in the coronary arteries, from growing. The information relayed to us suggested the patient was stable and the transport would be straightforward. This information later proved to be inaccurate, as he now required a high level of oxygen, was breathing twice the normal rate, and deteriorating rapidly.

The Transport:

The patient's room sat beyond where the nurses and doctor sit. Since the patient had been reported as stable, I decided to get report while my partner went to our patient's room. My discussion with the sending physician indicated the patient was doing well. Midway through our conversation, though, I noticed my partner walking out of the room, nodding his head, cluing me to get over there. I walked in his

159

direction and he whispered "you better come here." When I looked in the room, I thought *this guy should have been flown.*

In the bed lay an unresponsive, skinny, and chronically ill elderly man. He appeared malnourished and frail, had part of one leg amputated, and had infected ulcers on his only foot. His respiratory rate doubled the norm and his oxygen levels were critically low. Healthy young adults' oxygen saturations are normally over 95% and often 100%. His saturation was 80%. Many times this problem can be improved by placing an oxygen mask on the patient, but he was already on a 100% non-rebreathing oxygen mask, the highest level of oxygen available without placing a breathing tube. His blood pressure was normal, but his heart beat way above normal in the 140 to 150 range. It was clear he wasn't leaving the emergency department without a breathing tube.

I hurried back to the nurses' station and asked if the patient's doctor and nurse might come to the room. Both the doctor and nurse followed me back and looked surprised that the patient had deteriorated so much. We discussed flying the patient, but because of a construction problem with the helipad, a helicopter could not land there. The alternate landing zone for this hospital was 10 minutes away. Regardless of the patient's condition, he would have to travel by a mobile ICU for at least part of the transport. The hospital he was going to is a 15 or 20 minute drive, so calling an aircraft at this point would not save any time and, in fact, would delay his transfer quite a bit. Since our crew is the same crew who staffs the aircraft, only on a mobile ICU this day, we proceeded with the transport.

We all agreed that placing a breathing tube before we left was the right thing to do for the patient and I asked if they would help with the intubation. My partner had already gotten everything needed out to place the tube and began to draw up the medications to sedate and paralyze our patient. Sometimes, giving sedation can lower blood pressure and lead to other complications, especially if the patient has poor cardiac function. None of us knew his cardiac history, but based on his other illnesses and his current blood tests we assumed he had prior heart attacks along with a weak heart. Since the patient was unresponsive, and we didn't want to drop his blood pressure inadvertently, the physician and I agreed to try the intubation without sedation.

I moved to the head of the bed, and without giving sedation, removed his oxygen mask and tried to open his mouth. As I inserted my index finger into his mouth, he clamped his teeth shut. I put the oxygen mask back on our patient and my partner gave a small dose of sedation. Next, I put a different type of mask on our patient, allowing me to breathe for him as he drifted off to sleep. While the sedation began to work, I manually ventilated him with an ambu bag.

Once he was asleep, I again inserted my finger into his mouth, this time a bit more slowly to make sure he didn't clamp his teeth on my finger. I opened his mouth and inserted a laryngoscope to look for his vocal cords. As soon as I peered in, the cords came into clear site, opening and closing as he subconsciously attempted to breathe. I waited for them to open, and placed the tube through the cords and into the trachea.

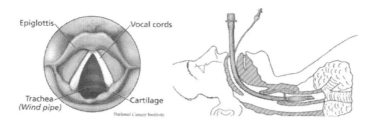

We verified it was in the proper location and squeezed several breaths of oxygen into his lungs. Seconds later, his oxygen levels improved to normal and a tremendous sense of relief came over me. We secured the tube and assigned ventilation duties to the respiratory therapist while we prepared to leave.

We thought the challenging part of the transport was behind us, since we had now secured our patients airway, and we rechecked his vital signs. His oxygen levels remained normal and his heart rate was improving, but his blood pressure had dropped: it was now only 74/42. Systolic blood pressures (top number) of 90 to 100 are considered "low-normal" and 74 was too low.

Hypotension, or low blood pressure, is not uncommon after getting sedation for intubation, and although concerned, we were not excessively worried. Provided the low blood pressure is corrected rather quickly, little harm is caused by the brief episode. However, if the pressure remains low for a prolonged period complications can develop, so we gave intravenous (IV) fluid wide open to correct it. This is known as a fluid bolus and the goal of this is to fill the intravascular space with volume to increase the blood pressure. Often with a fluid bolus, and as the sedation wears off, the hypotension resolves within minutes.

Even though we expected his blood pressure to return to normal, we mixed an IV medication called norepinephrine to increase his pressure in case the fluid we gave did not work. We checked the pressure again, but it hadn't improved much: it was now 76/42. We had to fix this before other complications developed, so we started the norepinephrine IV infusion, and within minutes, his blood pressure had returned to normal. He appeared to be stable and we felt comfortable in proceeding with transport. I took the ambu bag from the respiratory therapist and we left the bedside, loaded the patient into the mobile ICU, and connected him to our transport ventilator. The events that would soon transpire while in the ambulance are moments in my life I will never forget.

We rechecked his blood pressure several times, and things seemed stable until midway through the trip. We had placed an end tidal carbon dioxide ($ETCO_2$) monitor, which connects between the ventilator tubing and breathing tube. This allowed us to monitor our ventilation and make sure we were adequately breathing for our patient. The $ETCO_2$ will show the level of carbon dioxide (CO_2) that comes from the blood and is blown off by the lungs through the breathing tube.

Normally, the CO_2 rises if you are not bagging at fast enough rates, or the ventilator breath rate is set to slow to remove the CO_2 in the body. We were able to monitor this with the $ETCO_2$ monitor, but what does it mean if it drops rapidly? Well, equipment problems aside, you might be bagging too fast or the ventilator might be breathing too fast and blowing off too much CO_2. These are the most common reasons but there could be something else going on with the patient. If the heart isn't moving blood past the lungs, it can't bring the CO_2 from the body, and you end up moving the same gas back and forth through the tube. This is exactly what happened. Out of nowhere, his $ETCO_2$ declined without warning.

Attempting to find the reason for the sudden decline, we recycled our blood pressure cuff and verified the tube was in place by listening for his lung sounds. My partner disconnected our patient from the ventilator and began to manually ventilate with the ambu bag. I listened with a stethoscope over his chest and heard air movement, so I knew the breathing tube was still in the right place. By this time there was no blood pressure reading, so I felt for a radial pulse near his wrist but it was not there.

My partner and I both moved to check the carotid pulse in the neck, but it, too, had disappeared. We had a heart rhythm on the monitor but no pulse. We increased our norepinephrine IV infusion and began cardiopulmonary resuscitation (CPR) for pulseless electrical activity (PEA). There was an electrical heart rhythm but his heart did not pump effectively: the goal of our chest compressions was to circulate blood throughout the body.

CPR in the hospital with a multitude of resources is quite a task itself. Imagine doing this with 2 people in a bouncing ambulance while going down the highway with lights and sirens. I gave chest compressions while my partner drew up and gave advanced cardiac life support medications and gave a breath every few seconds. We continued CPR and alternated chest compression duties, pausing every 2 minutes to briefly feel for a pulse, but we never found one.

I yelled to the driver to call our destination and inform them of the situation and tell them that we would now be going straight to the emergency department (ED). Within a few minutes, we arrived at the hospital and diverted to the ED. With CPR still in progress, we placed the patient on their bed and continued to help the hospital staff with CPR.

The Outcome:

After 10 more minutes of CPR and several advanced cardiac life support medications, we regained a pulse. The patient was then transferred to the ICU. Unfortunately, he had no neurological recovery and his family withdrew care several days later. I replayed this transport many times that day, week, and month, wondering what else I might have done or if I missed anything that may have contributed to his demise.

Take Home Points:

For the Nurse or EMS Provider:

Look at your patient as soon as possible, before report, because things can change in an instant. I didn't at least peak in the room before taking report and assumed everything was okay.

End tidal CO_2 monitoring – In this transport, before we checked for a pulse or blood pressure we noticed his $ETCO_2$ dropped to single digits and this clued us to the fact he might be in cardiac arrest. Once we began chest compressions, his $ETCO_2$ did rise slightly because we moved blood past the lungs. If $ETCO_2$ drops, troubleshoot the device, but consider the possibility that the heart might not be moving blood.

When we first assessed our patient – his oxygen level was in the low 80s with a good waveform (pleth) on the monitor and he was breathing 35-40 times a minute. He could have been breathing fast either from a lack of oxygen or a severe acidosis caused by a lack of perfusion or both. He was likely trying to blow off excess CO_2, and although we tried to ventilate him at a higher than normal rate, we may not have ventilated him at a fast enough rate, which may have contributed to his acidosis.

An arterial line in this patient would have been useful and I regret not placing one. We may have been able to identify an acute drop in blood pressure quicker and treat it sooner.

For the Public:

Although this was not a good outcome, CPR has saved a countless number of lives, and I have performed CPR on many patients who survived and went on to live productive and long lives. I encourage everyone to learn it.

CPR should be performed until professionals arrive and generally is:

- 30 chest compressions to the heart followed by two resuscitation breaths (goal is 100-120 compressions per minute).
- Many health care professionals now say that mouth to mouth breathing may not be necessary and only compressions can be done.

GUATEMALA AND BACK, THAT'S A LONG TRANSPORT

Flight Nurses never know where they will be, whom they might meet, when they'll get home, and/or what interesting patients they may wind up transporting. On one particular day in March of 2012, little did I know I would be taking a trip to Guatemala City in Guatemala, Mexico. Nor did I know that I would not arrive home until some 22 hours later, the following day. Up until this point in my career I had flown on many fixed-wing (i.e. "airplane") missions, but never outside the continental United States. This transport would prove to be one I will never forget.

0700

Scheduled to fly in a helicopter this day, I had just finished checking the equipment to make sure everything was in order. I was asked if I would fly to Guatemala on a special Very Important Person (VIP) mission. The flight was scheduled to take 4.5 hours each way. We would leave in 2 hours and fly nonstop both ways. At this point it was 7:45 AM and I thought to myself: *Well, if we are in the air by 10:00 or 11:00 AM, we'll arrive in Guatemala at around 3:30 PM, be on the ground for an hour or so, and back in the air by 5:00 PM. This would put me home around 10:00 or 11:00 PM.* I had always wanted to take a mission out of the country and this was my chance. With this in mind, I thought that even though it would be later than normal, I'd still be home at a decent hour.

0800

Before agreeing to the mission, I called my wife and asked her opinion about my leaving the country and coming home late. I had arrived home late several days in a row that same week and knew she wanted me home for some overdue family time. Being the dedicated and understanding wife she is, she sensed I wanted to go on the mission and agreed. She seemed somewhat worried about me going so far, so I tried to reassure her and said I would text message her as much as possible from our work mobile phone. To tell the truth, though, I didn't know if the phone would even work out of the country, and because of that I told her not to worry if I didn't contact her.

After getting the okay from my wife, I agreed to the transport. Everything was set and instead of flying on a helicopter, I would now be going to Guatemala on a plane. One small problem existed, though. I had left my passport at home, not expecting to leave the country that morning. I thought that since we did not leave for another 2 hours, I would run home, get my passport, and drive right to the airport. I told the trip coordinator I needed to hurry home and get my passport, and I would meet up with the other crew-member flying with me at the airport. My unexpected trip to Guatemala would prove to be the first of many surprises that day.

Not long after agreeing to the mission, the coordinator received a patient status update and discovered the patient needed a ventilator and a high oxygen requirement. He needed two intravenous (IV) infusions, one of which was a controlled substance used for sedation called lorazepam, also known as Ativan. He had also been getting a paralytic on occasion to aid with ventilation. This man sounded sick and the transport might be challenging and I thought: *what have I managed to get myself into?* Our transport drug bag only carries a small supply of these medications and we did not have an adequate amount for this long of a trip. We needed to get enough of these medications to safely complete the transport.

After an hour of talking with our pharmacy and obtaining several required signatures, we obtained the needed drugs. This included ten vials of a paralytic called Vecuronium, two IV bags of lorazepam, and two IV bags of the pain medication fentanyl. These medications are controlled substances, so I could no longer simply place them in my car and drive straight to the airport as planned. I would have to instead return so security personnel could escort me to the airport with the medications and narcotics. Although this created an inconvenience, we now had enough medications to safely complete our mission, so I left for my house, got my passport, and returned at around 10:00 AM.

1000

In the hour it took me to drive home and obtain my passport, somehow our flight plans changed, and we were no longer flying nonstop to Guatemala. The crew flying the plane based at the airport did not have enough duty time to legally fly both ways. This meant we now needed to fly to Florida and meet up with another crew, who would in turn fly us to Guatemala and then back home.

At this point I recognized I'd be home much later than I anticipated and became somewhat reluctant to go on what would now be a very long trip. I had committed to going on the flight, though. Besides, I knew the coordinators would not be able to find another team member who was willing to make the trip and who had a passport on their person. This did not look to be a routine trip, either, given the fact he was on a ventilator, had a high oxygen requirement, and needed several IV infusions. Most importantly, the flight was slated to lift within an hour. This reality, coupled with the fact that the trip would be out of the country, made prospects for another flight team virtually impossible.

There was no backing out, and I moved forward with the mission. Hospital security personnel accompanied and drove us to the airport where our fixed wing equipment is located. On the way I sent a text message to my wife to update her about the delay and that I would be home later than planned. I told her I loved her, for her not to worry, and that I would contact her as much as possible throughout the trip.

1100

I arrived at the airport and went through our various medical bags several times to make sure everything was in order. In addition to these bags, I made sure we had a patient monitor, ventilator, batteries and power cords, ECG wires and stickers, extra working IV pumps (needed in case one should fail), and a portable oxygen tank. Everything was stocked with the right amount of equipment. All the gear had been checked and was in good working condition. We had the extra medications obtained from our pharmacy and all appeared ready for our departure, so I loaded everything into the plane.

The pilots flying us to Florida were likewise ready and briefed us on the upcoming flight. I had one final thought before we left. I thought it might be worthwhile to bring the largest portable oxygen tank we can carry. While somewhat awkward to move, it might not only prove useful but perhaps even vital late in the trip. We were airborne and bound for Florida around noon. On the flight, I reviewed the internal oxygen consumption calculator on our transport ventilator to make sure I'd be able to estimate oxygen use during transport.

1430

We landed in sunny Florida, and to our delight, we found the plane we would be taking to Guatemala waiting on us. I walked to the awaiting plane to check out the inside of the aircraft. I had never flown in this particular aircraft before and wanted to familiarize myself with its environment. The cabin was a bit larger than most medical aircraft yet much smaller than that of a commercial airliner. Its interior was almost 6 feet wide, 20 feet long, and 5 feet high. Not even enough room inside for a grown person to stand. I went through the normal checklists for this plane to ensure transport readiness. All was adequate in the aircraft, but we had one small dilemma.

The plane did carry one of the largest oxygen tanks available (i.e. an "M tank"), but it only had a pressure of 1900 PSI with a full capacity of 2200 PSI. For 99% of the flights we fly, 1900 PSI would be a more than ample amount of oxygen to handle virtually any emergency. This would also last over 22 hours with a patient on a nasal cannula, a fairly low oxygen supply often seen in the hospital; however, our patient required much more. With the tank only 85% full, there was room for more oxygen, so I asked our pilots if it might be topped-off. They informed me it could be, but indicated it might take an hour-and-a-half to do so because of mechanical issues with the oxygen truck. I almost said to myself not to worry about it to avoid further delay, but I knew the patient needed high oxygen therapy and my better judgment dictated we top-off the tank so as not to risk running out of oxygen. Consequently, this delayed us an additional 1.5 hours.

The oxygen arrived and we departed Florida destined for Guatemala two hours after landing. Before departing, though, our new pilots informed us that when we landed it would be rush hour and to expect a long transport time to the hospital. I might add, the family of our patient had generously offered us their helicopter, but it lacked the needed medical equipment. Moreover, I was not about to get into an aircraft, in a foreign country, operated by a company I knew nothing about. Just before our departure, I sent a final text to my wife telling her I loved her and shut my phone off to avoid any potential global service charges. A final reassuring thought entered my mind after learning of the potential long ground transport: *I'm glad I brought the largest portable oxygen tank we have.*

1945-On the ground in Guatemala

We landed in Guatemala around 7:45 PM, faced with a long ground transport time ahead of us. We originally had planned to be headed back home by this time. I turned on the company mobile phone and, to my pleasant surprise, the phone worked. I had just sent a quick text to my wife and informed her we had landed in Guatemala safely when we were confronted with yet another delay. Customs officials

174

informed us they needed to inspect our equipment before we would be able to leave our plane. Dressed in military gear, they carried what looked to be machine guns hanging from their necks, and proceeded to board our plane and ask for our passports. For the first time on this journey, I realized I was no longer in my home country and that I couldn't leave whenever I desired. The custom officials spoke in my direction but all I understood was "paramedico, paramedico" and I nodded my head in the affirmative. After what seemed to be a 15-minute interrogation, they allowed us to depart from the plane.

It was now dark outside. I got off the aircraft and noticed what looked to be a minivan with emergency lights on it. We were transporting an important figure in Guatemala and many assistants had been arranged to help with the transport. Although much appreciated, all the help was not necessary. One of the assistants happened to be the patient's cousin, who thankfully spoke English. Not being able to speak Spanish, I could only communicate with my partner and the cousin, so I asked him if I could look inside the ambulance. I peeked in the squad and noticed two rather small oxygen tanks and said to myself: *damn, that's not enough oxygen.* These tanks would probably last a total of twenty to thirty minutes at best. Further complicating the problem was the fact that our ventilator could not connect to their oxygen because of different connection fittings. The only way possible for us to access this oxygen would be to connect to an ambu bag and then manually ventilate the patient.

I asked the cousin who spoke English how long it would take to drive to the hospital. He informed me that, because of rush hour, the ride there would normally last from 45-60 minutes, but noted that since we would be accompanied by a police escort, the drive might only take 20 or 25 minutes. I figured that with the spare tank I had brought, plus the two small ambulance oxygen tanks, we just might be able to get back to the airport with enough oxygen provided there were no delays. Had we been stateside in the U.S., I would have arranged for another ambulance and not taken any chances. Since that was not the case, and given our communication difficulties and the fact we had already been delayed, I moved forward with the transport. But we would have to try to lower his oxygen use and totally paralyze the patient to avoid wasting any vitally needed oxygen.

The ride to the hospital was unlike any I had ever experienced. Six police escorted us to the hospital, riding off-road motorcycles with lights flashing and sirens screaming. Traffic was bumper to bumper, horns screamed as we weaved in and out of slow moving cars...continually stopping and going, turning left then turning right. I began to think to myself: *I don't know any of these people...I'm in a foreign country...we hardly have any oxygen...all this equipment is useless to us...and I'm transporting a very prominent patron of this country.* With these thoughts in mind I looked at my partner and asked, "What the hell did we get ourselves into?" He looked at me, nodded his head and said with a smile on his face, "I don't know." After what may best be described as a twenty-minute roller coaster ride we arrived at the hospital around 8:30 PM.

2030-At the hospital in Guatemala

Thirteen hours after I agreed to transport a patient from Guatemala to the United States I saw him for the very first time. Two other people at the hospital, aside from my partner and I, spoke English, one of which was the cousin who met us at the airport. Fortunately, the sending attending physician spoke both English and Spanish. We talked with the doc and obtained useful and valuable information about the patient, including the circumstances that led to his present condition.

Our patient had acute mitral valve regurgitation causing pulmonary edema. This meant that some of the blood normally pumping from the heart, out the aorta and then through the body, was now pumping back into his lungs. Fluid had accumulated in his lungs to the point that he developed extreme difficulty breathing, which in turn led to his overall deterioration and need for a breathing tube. To complicate things even further, all signs suggested he most likely also had pneumonia.

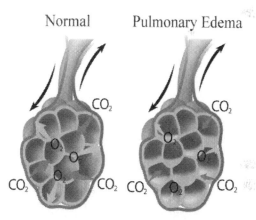

The reason he needed to be transported to a hospital in the United States was that he needed a mechanical valve replacement. In Guatemala at that time, they only put in "pig valves," which don't last as long as a mechanical valve. Since this was a relatively young man, the consensus of opinion thought he might survive the transport. Once in the U.S., the mechanical valve replacement procedure could be performed. Neither the transport nor the procedure would be without inherent risk, though.

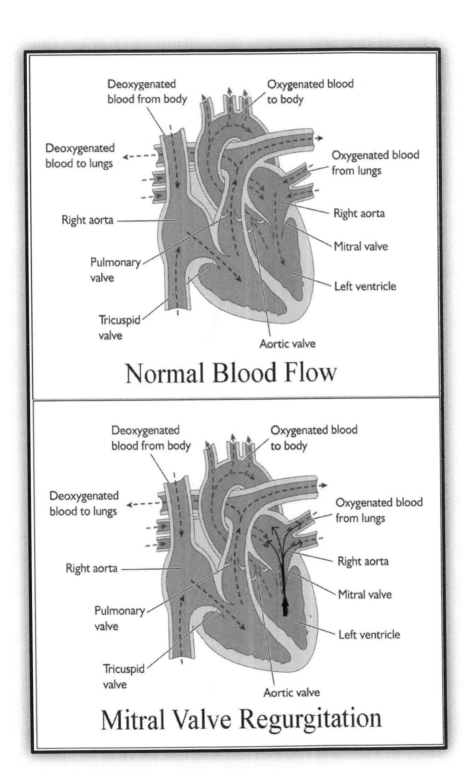

Normal Blood Flow

Mitral Valve Regurgitation

178

A mechanical mitral valve replacement seemed to be our patient's best option for definitive treatment, but that would not happen until after we transported him stateside. In the interim, we needed to manage his current condition and keep him alive until the procedure could be done. The goal for this condition in almost every instance is to lower the pressure in the aorta. In doing this, blood will flow in the path of least resistance and hopefully travel to the body and not the lungs. The sending facility had been attempting to do this with a nitroglycerin IV infusion. Many institutions prefer to do this intervention with other drugs such as sodium nitroprusside, but the nitro was a decent choice for our patient and appeared to be working so we kept it going. In transport, maintaining things as they are is sometimes challenging enough.

Not able to communicate verbally with any of the nurses, I hand signaled that we would roll the patient over on his side and put a "Reaves stretcher" under him while he was still on the bed. This is a flexible stretcher, similar to a strong tarp with handles, often supported by wooden planks. With this stretcher under him, any needed future movements of the patient would be much easier. After many hand signals, we placed the stretcher under our patient and then attached him to our monitoring equipment. I secured our oxygen tank between his legs to avoid messing around with it later. Because we had a limited supply, everything needed to be ready to go once we placed the patient on our portable tank.

The concentrations of medications for our Guatemalan patient were different than those found in the U.S. This created an additional step when calculating the IV infusion rates on the IV pumps. My calculations suggested that if we continued the nitro at the same dose, we had enough to complete the mission. I moved to the other IV infusion and noticed a drug labeled midazolam. This became a problem because we had been told our patient was on lorazepam, which was one of the extra drugs we had brought. These two drugs work similarly, but it takes longer for the sedating effects of lorazepam to take effect and one never knows for certain how a patient will respond to a particular medication. In this situation, though, we had no choice other than to use lorazepam. At our patient's current midazolam infusion rate, and given our existing stock supply, we would have run out within an hour. Consequently, we started our lorazepam infusion at an estimated equivalent dosage, knowing full well we would likely have to make medication adjustments. We also started an infusion of fentanyl to eliminate any potential pain our patient might have been experiencing, not to mention, it would give a desired side effect of sedation.

We secured the monitor at an angle between the patient's legs in a direction that allowed us to see our patient's vital signs once inside the aircraft. This prevented the need and wasted effort of manipulating the monitor during the flight. We positioned the monitor next to the oxygen tank, secured a foley catheter to the opposite leg, and attached our 3 IV pumps to the monitor. Then we fastened the stretcher straps around it all, making sure everything was in place and nothing would shift when we moved him. All these wires, lines, and tubing looked like spaghetti. Nevertheless, we did our best to keep everything in proper order. After all was secured, we moved our transport cot next to the bed while keeping the patient on the hospital ventilator to conserve as much oxygen as possible. We then lifted the Reeves Stretcher, with all our equipment secured in one bundle, onto the ambulance cot.

We were next confronted with an important issue at a crucial moment during transport. How would our patient tolerate being on our ventilator? In some circumstances it's possible, maybe even advisable, to manually vent a patient. Frankly, I have manually vented patients for a considerable length of time because they did not tolerate a transport ventilator. In this instance, though, the trip would be far too long in duration to try this. We expected to need our hands for other duties and needed the ventilator to work.

I wanted to check our patient's vital signs while on our ventilator, but didn't want to waste our limited supply of oxygen. Once on our oxygen, I intended for us to leave the hospital immediately to improve the likelihood of arriving at the airport without running out. I went to connect our ventilator oxygen hose to the hospital oxygen supply only to find these connections different and not compatible with each other. Although likely not an FDA "approved" method, I found a way to "MacGyver" or "jury-rig" a connection to the hospital oxygen supply. This seemed to work and we then placed him on our ventilator using their oxygen. At about this time, the patient began to wake up due to the changes we made in his sedation meds. This required us to increase our doses of both sedation (lorazepam) and pain (fentanyl) medication. We also tried to lower his oxygen requirement in an effort to conserve it. Seconds after doing this, though, his oxygen levels dropped abruptly, forcing us to put him back on the level he had previously been at.

We were still faced with figuring out the right sedation dosage. Our patient began to awaken again, breathing at too fast of a rate. This might be problematic once on our tank because each breath our patient took would lower our oxygen supply, even if only slightly. If these high rates continued, we would arrive at the airport with little or no oxygen remaining in our portable tank. Without oxygen, our patient might die. We again increased his sedation, and this time we gave a paralytic to entirely control each breath he took.

The paralytic took effect within minutes and after an hour at our patient's bedside, medically he appeared stable. His breathing had now slowed to a normal rate. Feeling comfortable with our patient's current status, we connected our ventilator to the portable oxygen tank situated between his legs and departed beside. We left the hospital, loaded our patient into the ambulance, and then proceeded to drive back to the airport in Guatemala. No matter what happened from this point, our destination was back to the airport and then home. Should any complications arise, we would manage them to the best of our ability with the equipment and medications we had.

2130-The ambulance ride back to the airport in Guatemala

The ride back to the airport seemed as brutal as the ride from there. We preferred a slow and smooth transport back to the airport, but if we did this, our oxygen might run out. All we could do was make sure everything stayed secure and pray. I distinctly remember thinking to myself: *what if something goes wrong...what would I do?* Here we were in a foreign country, with a high-level patient, managing his care. Should something go wrong: *how would they react...would I get back home...would they think it was our fault?* These are questions I'm grateful I'll never know the answer to. Although rough, the ride to the airport proved to be uneventful, and as it turned out, we had a quarter (¼) tank of oxygen remaining when we pulled onto the tarmac. Because of the larger portable oxygen tank we had brought, we didn't have to resort to manually bagging the patient and using the ambulance's comparatively small oxygen supply. I was so glad I had brought that tank.

2150-Back at the airport in Guatemala

Once back at the airport in Guatemala, we found customs officials still waiting for us in their military gear. But every minute that ticked by lowered our oxygen level and if forced to go through another long inspection, we might run out. I told this to both the translator and a family member, who in turn said something to one of the officials, who then expedited the inspection.

We parked inside a hangar at the airport and noticed about 15 people waiting inside to bid farewell to their friend. After a quick but needed bathroom break, we loaded our patient into the plane with 200 PSI (1/10th) remaining on our portable oxygen tank. As soon as we boarded, we connected to the aircraft oxygen supply. Overall, everything appeared much improved now. Our ventilator was now connected to one of the largest mobile oxygen supply sources available, a full M tank, and we were heading home. We secured everything in the aircraft and made sure the patient was stable in preparation for a 4.5 hour flight home. I simply can't express how relieved I was, knowing we were heading home.

Both the patient's wife and his brother accompanied us back to the U.S., so the plane was a bit cramped. We had not eaten for several hours and our patient's cousin had graciously bought us hamburgers. Now it was almost 10:00 PM. I scarfed down my sandwich and checked the company phone as we taxied down the runway. By this time my wife had text messaged me several times wondering if I was okay. As we lifted, I sent her a text message to inform her I was headed home, not sure it even went through before losing a signal.

2200-The flight back home from Guatemala

We reached cruising altitude, where the air is thinner and patients often need more oxygen. During the transition to 35,000 ft., we continued to monitor our patient's vital signs, and his oxygen level dropped, indicating he wasn't getting enough. We had no choice but to increase the oxygen percentage to keep him alive, realizing, of course, this also meant we would run out sooner. The other options were to ask our pilots to pressurize the cabin or descend to lower altitude. Either of these, however, would increase our flight time and the result would be the same - we still might run out of oxygen. Rather than lengthen the flight time, we elected to keep our current altitude and continue to closely monitor our oxygen status. I used functions on the ventilator to estimate how much time we had before running out. These calculations suggested that with an expected 4.5 hour flight, we would land with approximately 200-300 PSI (1/10th) oxygen remaining in the aircraft tank and only 200 PSI remaining in the portable tank I had brought. Man, this might be close.

When flying into the United States from another country, altering course apparently isn't the easiest thing to do and stopping to obtain more oxygen would cause another long delay. So it became necessary to prevent our patient from waking up and becoming anxious, because he would breathe too rapidly, expending vitally needed oxygen. In order to prevent this from occurring, every time our patient showed the slightest sign he was waking up we increased his sedation and administered another dose of paralytic. I remember administering 7 or 8 doses of the paralytic alone during the transport. In effect we were sedating, paralyzing, and then titrating our patient's blood pressure medication the entire 4.5 hour flight. Every 10 minutes, I eyeballed the oxygen gauge and calculated how much our patient had used, afraid we might run out. Halfway into the flight, it looked as if the oxygen supply would hold out provided nothing unexpected happened. Every so often I would make my way to the front of the aircraft to check our estimated time of arrival (ETA). We began our descent to land with 400 PSI left in the oxygen tank and it looked like we were home free.

0230 the next day-back on the ground in the U.S

We landed back home in the United States, a U.S. Customs official boarded our plane, and we explained to him our oxygen situation. Thankfully, he expedited the inspection and we unloaded the patient from the aircraft, placed him into an awaiting ambulance with a full M tank, and connected to their oxygen supply. We then drove to the hospital he had been accepted to and administered one final paralytic on the way. Although we now had plenty of oxygen, we wanted to avoid any potential problems for the final 15 minutes of the journey. We took our patient to his intensive care room, placed him on the bed, and removed our equipment while he was simultaneously placed on the hospital monitor, ventilator, and IV pumps.

The trip was a success and now our patient would hopefully survive his surgery. I knew in my heart I had done all I could for our patient and felt quite a sense of accomplishment with everything we had done. The ambulance took us back to the airport where we restocked all our equipment so it was ready to go for the next team. As much as I wanted to just go home and not restock all we had used, a responsible life flight team is never finished until all is ready for the next mission. When it's time for a life flight mission, everything must be ready to go in a moment's notice. Finally, I arrived home at 4:30 in the morning to find my wife sound asleep with her phone on her chest.

The Outcome:

Several days later I flew by helicopter to the institution he had his surgery. He had the mitral valve repair and was in a recovery unit, so I went to see how he was doing. I spoke with his wife and met several other members of his family whom I recalled seeing while in Guatemala. They told me their loved one still thought he was in Mexico. Understandably, he was confused at that point, so I didn't talk with him. Instead, I saw him several days later. He stayed in the hospital for several weeks but made a full recovery.

He personally wanted to thank me and we met for lunch one afternoon before he flew back home. This was one of the most rewarding moments in my career. I asked him if he remembered anything about his trip and he said the only thing he remembered was feeling like he was waking up in the middle of the ocean, drowning underwater, and trying to swim to air above. I felt awful he had that recollection but it made sense given the medical problems he experienced. Looking back, I wonder if the movements he made during the flight, the same movements we tried to stop, were the swimming movements he spoke of in his dream.

THE END

ABOUT THE AUTHOR

David M. Kaniecki MSN, ACNP-C, RN, CCRN is an acute care nurse practitioner (ACNP) for the Cleveland Clinic Critical Care Transport Team. He is responsible for the management of acute and chronically ill patients requiring transport via helicopter, fixed wing, or ground ambulance. He earned an Associate Degree in Nursing from North Central State College in 2005 and completed a Master of Science in Nursing (MSN) program at Case Western Reserve University (CWRU) in 2012 where he is now pursuing his Doctorate of Nursing Practice (DNP). At CWRU, he has maintained a 4.0 GPA and was awarded the 2012 Cushing-Robb Scholarship for excellence in academic achievement, clinical nursing ability, and professional competence.

He has practiced in a variety of critical care settings and cared for patients of multiple disease pathologies. Before becoming an ACNP, he worked as a staff nurse in a surgical intensive care unit (ICU), medical ICU, neurological ICU, cardiovascular ICU, coronary ICU and ICU float pool. With the skills acquired from his experience in the inpatient hospital setting, in 2008 he became a flight transport nurse to practice in unorthodox environments and has transported patients needing extreme levels of life support to a higher level of care both in the United States and globally. David has worked to share his knowledge and experience with student nurses as a nursing lab instructor and used his clinical experience for healthcare innovation. He is the inventor of a method and device to improve safety and accuracy in hemodynamic monitoring and is now working to bring this new technology to a world market.

Mr. Kaniecki is a member of the American Association of Critical Care Nurses (AACN) and holds many certifications and credentials including: Board Certified Acute Care Nurse Practitioner, Board Certified Registered Nurse, CCRN (Critical Care Registered Nurse), Advanced Trauma Life Support, Advanced Cardiac Life Support, Pediatric Advanced Life Support, Neonatal Resuscitation, Basic Life Support, and is NIH Stroke Scale Certified.

Path to a Nursing Career

David has transported more than patients across the United States. After graduating from Ashland High School in 1993, he worked on a farm and drove a tractor-trailer for a small family owned business called Mitchell and Sons Moving & Storage. There he spent almost 7 years of his life both farming and transporting household goods. He transitioned to a second truck driving job, and shortly after his employment with this company began, an incident at that job would change his life forever.

David's path to nursing, and later a nurse practitioner, started in 2002 at a truck stop in Indiana. At that time, in his mid-20s and an over-the-road truck driver, he believed his life had a higher meaning. On his way home from a trucking road trip, he stopped at a truck stop in Indiana. There he fueled his truck, parked, and walked inside to use the restroom. In the restroom he noticed an unconscious elderly man lying on the bathroom floor. Although unsure of what to do, he had seen cardiopulmonary resuscitation (CPR) on television and attempted chest compressions and rescue breaths. He yelled to the teller working that day to call 911, pulled the unconscious man out of the restroom, and performed CPR until help came. A squad arrived in minutes, took over CPR, and later revived the elderly man. From that point forward, David wanted the skills and knowledge to save the lives of others.

After this event, he searched for employment at several fire departments wanting to become a paramedic, and in the meantime, continued to drive a tractor-trailer. Within months of the incident at the truck stop, fate intervened. The company he had been driving for decided to outsource their shipping department. He was given an option to continue employment with the new company, but instead chose to return to school. Realizing a nursing degree would provide more career opportunities than a paramedic, he obtained an associate degree in nursing and chose to specialize in critical care, where he continues to love his profession.

A FINAL THOUGHT ON AIR MEDICAL SAFETY

Helicopter Emergency Medical Service (HEMS): We know how to improve safety; we just won't pay for it

Helicopter Emergency Medical Service (HEMS) programs have one of the highest fatality rates per employee than any other occupation and are 6000 times more likely to have an accident than commercial aircraft. We ask HEMS crews to transport our loved ones in times of their greatest need yet continue to allow them to be governed by a different set of safety rules than those very aircraft we fly in. The primary reason safety improvements have not been made is because of the little financial reward for aircraft vendors to invest in safety. America should require the same safety equipment for HEMS services as we do the commercial aircraft we fly in. Since HEMS aircraft vendors are unlikely to receive additional safety funding when healthcare is trying to reduce spending, those who triage patients for flight must be aware of the risks and costs to avoid unnecessary flights.

Any commercial aircraft carrying over 10 passengers is required to fly with two pilots and have substantially lower accident rates than HEMS yet less than 1% of HEMS are dual pilot operations. Do these flight nurses, medics and doctors not deserve the same level of safety as commercial fliers? The FAA, in 2009, published 9 recommendations to help improve the safety for HEMS crews resulting in only one mandate or regulatory change in HEMS operations. Most of the proposed recommendations involve the use and implementation of more sophisticated equipment imposing a higher workload on the pilot which may require additional manpower to operate. Pilots with a high mental workload and auditory input experience considerable difficulty in carrying out primary operation tasks [6].

There is minimal financial incentive for an HEMS vendor to purchase or equip their aircraft with the cutting-edge technology or fly dual pilot operations. Some of the more sophisticated helicopters can cost upwards of $10-12 million dollars, however, an aircraft which seats only a single pilot and equipped with minimal safety equipment might by purchased for $1-3 million. In addition to costs required to purchase aircraft, paying one pilot is more cost effective than flying with two. HEMS vendors looking to be profitable are forced to cut costs to maximize profits because Medicare reimbursement rates are the same for all air medical transport companies regardless of the overhead costs.

We know the areas in which we need to improve yet little has been done to truly solve the problem. The opportunities for improvement have already been identified by the FAA but no real change is on the horizon unless dollars can be found to support the investment. America is in the process of reassessing where to best spend healthcare dollars. Unfortunately, until HEMS vendors are mandated to comply with FAA recommendations, only a select few companies will offer safer and more sophisticated aircraft, primarily because their contractor requires it.

If there is no legislative solution to improve the safety of HEMS aircraft, there is something healthcare can do to limit the risk exposure to HEMS crews by flying only patients who require rapid air transportation. Literature on the appropriate use of helicopter emergency medical services is controversial. Overuse of helicopters has been reported in approximately 85% of flights [7]. Bledsoe and colleagues reported a majority of trauma patients transported from scene accidents by helicopter have non-life-threatening injuries [8]. Other research shows more appropriate use of HEMS with only 1.3% of total flights determined to be inappropriate [9]. The true number is somewhere in the middle of those extremes but unnecessary HEMS flights occur daily in the U.S.

Appropriate triage is not taught in our medical or nursing schools nor is it stressed in healthcare's continuing education model. If we can't provide optimum safety conditions for our HEMS crews, the least we can do is educate those people who request HEMS services and limit unnecessary flights. Additionally, the credentialing bodies that allow these clinicians to practice should give credit to those providers who become educated in appropriate transport triage.

David M Kaniecki MSN, ACNP, CCRN

GLOSSARY OF TERMS

ABG - Arterial Blood Gas - An arterial blood gas (ABG) is a blood test that is performed using blood from an artery. It involves puncturing an artery with a thin needle and syringe and drawing a small volume of arterial blood. The most common puncture site is the radial artery at the wrist, but sometimes the femoral artery in the groin or other sites are used. The blood can also be drawn from an arterial catheter. An ABG is used to determine the pH of the blood, the partial pressure of carbon dioxide and oxygen, and the bicarbonate level.

Acidotic - Acidosis is an increased acidity in the blood. (i.e., an increased hydrogen ion concentration). It usually refers to acidity of the blood plasma. Acidosis is said to occur when arterial pH falls below 7.35, alkalosis occurs at a pH over 7.45.

Ambu Bag - An Ambu bag (also known as a bag valve mask or BVM) is a hand-held device used to provide positive pressure ventilation to a patient who is not breathing or who is breathing inadequately. Ambu bag is the proprietary name or is generically known as a manual resuscitator or "self-inflating bag". The full-form of AMBU is Artificial Manual Breathing Unit. The device is a standard part of a resuscitation kit for trained professionals. The BVM is frequently used in hospitals, and is a vital part of a crash cart. The device is widely used in the operating room to ventilate an anaesthetized patient in the minutes before a mechanical ventilator is attached. An Ambu Bag is self-filling with air, although additional oxygen is usually added by connecting it to an oxygen source.

Arterial line (A-line) - An arterial line is a thin catheter inserted into an artery. It is most commonly used in intensive care medicine to monitor the blood pressure in real-time, and to obtain samples for arterial blood gas measurements. An arterial line is usually inserted in the wrist (radial artery), elbow (brachial artery), or groin (femoral artery).

Bag Valve Mask - See Ambu Bag. These terms are often used interchangeably.

Bagging - Use of the Ambu Bag or BVM to ventilate a patient is often called "bagging" the patient. Bagging is frequently required in medical emergencies when the patient's breathing is insufficient (respiratory failure) or has ceased completely (respiratory arrest). The BVM resuscitator is used to manually provide mechanical ventilation in preference to mouth-to-mouth resuscitation.

BiPAP - BiPAP is an acronym for *bi-level positive airway pressure*. BiPAP is a method of respiratory ventilation that uses an oxygen delivery mask connected to a special machine. Oxygen delivery percentages can be increased with BiPAP. It's similar to CPAP but provides two levels of pressure: inspiratory positive airway pressure (IPAP) and a lower expiratory positive airway pressure (EPAP).

Bolus - The medical definition of bolus is the administration of a drug, medication or other substance in the form of a single, large dose. The term fluid bolus in this book refers to a large volume of intravenous fluid given rapidly.

Central Line – Term used for central venous catheter. This is a long, fine catheter introduced via a large vein into the superior vena cava or right atrium for administration of parenteral fluids or medications or for measurement of central venous pressure.

CO_2 - Molecular symbol for carbon dioxide.

CPAP - CPAP is an acronym for *continuous positive airway pressure*. CPAP is a method of respiratory ventilation that uses an oxygen delivery mask connected to a special machine. This machine blows air at a prescribed pressure. Oxygen delivery percentages can be increased with CPAP. It was initially used mainly by patients for the treatment of sleep apnea at home, but now is in widespread use across intensive care units as a form of ventilation.

Diastolic Blood Pressure - Diastolic blood pressure is the lower number in a blood pressure reading. It reflects the pressure in the arteries when the heart is relaxed.

Diuretic - A diuretic is any drug that elevates the rate of urination and thus provides a means to remove fluid from the body.

ETCO$_2$ (End Tidal Carbon Dioxide) - ETCO$_2$ refers to the level of carbon dioxide in air exhaled from the body. It's monitored with capnography and helps provide a rapid and reliable method to detect respiratory status and life-threatening conditions.

Fluid Bolus - see Bolus.

Intracranial - Intracranial refers to within the cranium.

Intubation - Intubation refers to endotracheal intubation. This is the insertion of a tube thru the mouth and into the trachea for purposes of anesthesia, airway maintenance, aspiration of secretions, lung ventilation, or prevention of entrance of foreign material into the airway.

Ischemia - Ischemia is an insufficient supply of blood to an organ, usually due to a blocked artery.

Laryngoscope - Laryngoscope is a medical device used to view the larynx. It can be used to facilitate visualization of vocal cords during intubation.

Murmur - Heart murmurs are extra heart sounds that are produced as a result of turbulent blood flow that is sufficient to produce audible noise. Most heart murmurs can only be heard with a stethoscope.

Nasal Cannula - A nasal cannula is a device used to deliver supplemental oxygen or airflow to a person in need of respiratory support. It cannot provide high concentrations of oxygen. This device consists of a plastic tube which fits behind the ears, and a set of two prongs which are placed in the nostrils. Oxygen flows from these prongs and into the nasal cavity. The nasal cannula is connected to an oxygen tank, a portable oxygen generator, or a wall connection in a hospital via a flowmeter.

Non-Rebreather - A non-rebreather mask (NRB) is a device used in medical emergencies that require oxygen therapy. An NRB requires that the patient can breathe unassisted, but unlike low flow nasal cannula, the NRB allows for the delivery of higher concentrations of oxygen.

Normal Vital Sign ranges for the average healthy adult:

- Blood pressure: 90/60 mm/Hg to 120/80 mm/Hg
- Breathing: 12 - 18 breaths per minute
- SpO_2 (oxygen saturation): >95% breathing room air
- Pulse: 60 - 100 beats per minute
- Temperature: 97.8 - 99.1 degrees Fahrenheit

O_2 - Molecular symbol for oxygen.

Occlusion - A coronary occlusion is the partial or complete obstruction of blood flow in a coronary artery. This often leads to a heart attack.

Palpable - Palpation is used as part of a physical examination in which an object is felt (usually with the hands of a healthcare practitioner). A palpable pulse is one that can be felt. If a pulse is non-palpable then it cannot be felt.

Perfuse - Perfuse refers to adequate blood flow. In medicine, it means to pass (a fluid) through organ tissue to ensure adequate exchange of oxygen and carbon monoxide.

Pressure Bag - A pressure bag is a device that is used to pressurize a bag filled with intravenous fluid for the purpose of regulating how quickly the fluid is dispensed to the patient. Pressure bags can help speed the rate of fluid delivery to patients.

STEMI - An ST-Elevation Myocardial Infarction (STEMI) is a life-threatening type of heart attack during which one of the heart's major arteries is blocked.

Systolic Blood Pressure - Systolic blood pressure is the higher or top number in a blood pressure reading. It reflects the pressure in the arteries when the heart contracts.

http://encyclopedia.thefreedictionary.com and http://en.wikipedia.org

Oxygen Delivery Devices

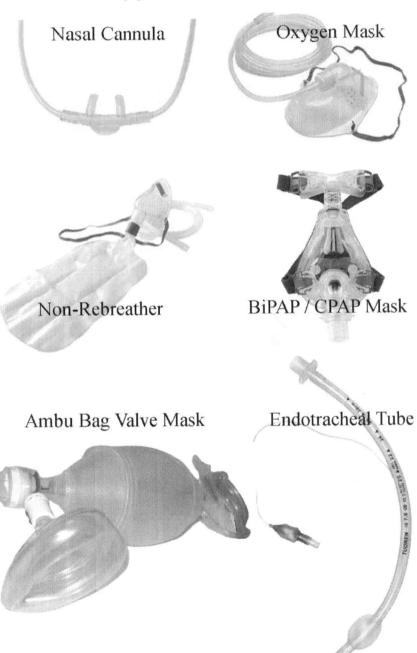

Nasal Cannula

Oxygen Mask

Non-Rebreather

BiPAP / CPAP Mask

Ambu Bag Valve Mask

Endotracheal Tube

REFERENCES

Miscellaneous works used: [10-13]

1. Warren J Manning, M., *Management of aortic dissection*, in *UpToDate*, M. Emile R Mohler III, et al., Editors. 2013.

2. Robert J Singer, M., M. Christopher S Ogilvy, and M. Guy Rordorf (2013) *Treatment of aneurysmal subarachnoid hemorrhage.*

3. UpToDate, *Furosemide: Drug information Lexicomp.* 2013.

4. Morgenstern, L.B., et al., *Guidelines for the management of spontaneous intracerebral hemorrhage: a guideline for healthcare professionals from the American Heart Association/American Stroke Association.* Stroke, 2010. **41**(9): p. 2108-29.

5. Abbas E Kitabchi, P., MD, FACP, FACE and M. Burton D Rose (2013) *Treatment of diabetic ketoacidosis and hyperosmolar hyperglycemic state in adults.*

6. Morris, C.H. and Y.K. Leung, *Pilot mental workload: how well do pilots really perform?* Ergonomics, 2006. **49**(15): p. 1581-96.

7. Moront, M.L., C.S. Gotschall, and M.R. Eichelberger, *Helicopter transport of injured children: system effectiveness and triage criteria.* J Pediatr Surg, 1996. **31**(8): p. 1183-6; discussion 1187-8.

8. Bledsoe, B.E., et al., *Helicopter scene transport of trauma patients with nonlife-threatening injuries: a meta-analysis.* J Trauma, 2006. **60**(6): p. 1257-65; discussion 1265-6.

9. Hafner, J.W., et al., *Inappropriate helicopter emergency medical services transports: results of a national cohort utilization review.* Prehosp Emerg Care, 2012. **16**(4): p. 434-42.

10. Dreamstime.com. 2013.

11. Bederson, J.B., et al., *Guidelines for the management of aneurysmal subarachnoid hemorrhage: a statement for healthcare professionals from a special writing group of the Stroke Council, American Heart Association.* Stroke, 2009. **40**(3): p. 994-1025.

12. TheFreeDictionary.com, *Medical dictionary.* 2013, Farlex, Inc. .

13. Wikipedia, t.f.e. 2013.

CONTRIBUTORS

Editor: Kate Frishman, RN, is a freelance copy editor who edits primarily in the nursing, scientific, business, and fiction fields - although she's always ready for a new challenge! She is also a hospice nurse, marriage officiant, and mother of five. She can be reached at katefrishman@gmail.com.

Reviewer: Gregory Ingram M.D.

Reviewer: James Kaniecki

Reviewer: AnnMarie Kaniecki

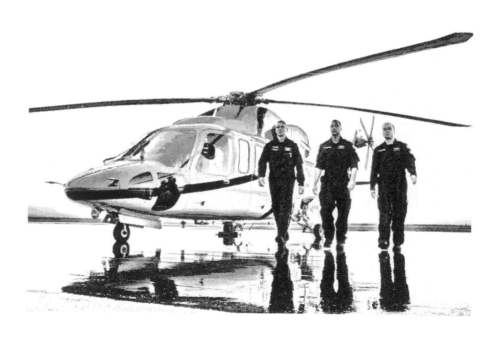

Made in the USA
Lexington, KY
06 August 2013